Pulmonary Function Tests in Clinical Practice

D0881957

Pulmonary Function Tests in Clinical Practice

Ali Altalag, Jeremy Road, and Pearce Wilcox

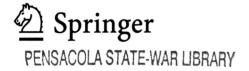

Springer

Ali Altalag, MD
Respirologist and Critical
Care Fellow
University of Toronto
Toronto General Hospital
585 University Ave, 11C-1170
Toronto, ON, M5G 2N2
Canada

Jeremy Road, MD
Professor of Medicine
University of British Columbia
Medical Director of Pulmonary
Function Lab
Vancouver General Hospital
2775 Laurel Street, 7th Floor
Vancouver, BC, V5Z 1M9
Canada

Pearce Wilcox, MD
Associate Professor of Medicine
University of British Columbia
Medical Director of Pulmonary
Function Lab
St. Paul's Hospital
1081 Burrard Street
Vancouver, BC, V6Z 1Y6
Canada

ISBN 978-1-84882-230-6   e-ISBN 978-1-84882-231-3
DOI 10.1007/978-1-84882-231-3

British Library Cataloguing in Publication Data
A catalogue record for this book is available from the British Library

Library of Congress Control Number:

© Springer-Verlag London Limited 2009
Apart from any fair dealing for the purposes of research or private study,
or criticism or review, as permitted under the Copyright, Designs and
Patents Act 1988, this publication may only be reproduced, stored or
transmitted, in any form or by any means, with the prior permission in
writing of the publishers, or in the case of reprographic reproduction in
accordance with the terms of licences issued by the Copyright Licensing
Agency. Enquiries concerning reproduction outside those terms should be
sent to the publishers.
The use of registered names, trademarks, etc. in this publication does not
imply, even in the absence of a specific statement, that such names are ex-
empt from the relevant laws and regulations and therefore free for general
use.
Product liability: The publisher can give no guarantee for information
about drug dosage and application thereof contained in this book. In every
individual case the respective user must check its accuracy by consulting
other pharmaceutical literature.

Printed on acid-free paper

springer.com

Preface

The volume of expelled air is believed to have been first measured by Galen in about 150 AD. However, it was not until the mid-1800s that Hutchinson designed a spirometer, very similar to the ones used today, which allowed routine measurement of exhaled lung volume. Finally, in 1969 Dubois designed the plethysmograph, which allowed a measure of the complete lung volume, which included the residual volume. Nowadays measuring spirometry has become routine with the advent of the pneumotachograph and computers. Although the technology is widely available and not excessive in cost, spirometry or the measurement of exhaled gas volume is still underutilized. To detect disease and assess its severity lung volume measures are extremely useful, indeed one might say mandatory, so the reason for this underutilization remains obscure. We hope that this book, which is aimed at the clinician, helps to explain the basics of lung volume measurement and hence increases its utility. The text also includes an overview of exercise and respiratory sleep diagnostic tests for the clinician.

Ali Altalag   *Toronto, ON*
Jeremy Road   *Vancouver, BC*
Pearce Wilcox   *Vancouver, BC*

Acknowledgements

We acknowledge everyone who helped in producing this book. A special acknowledgment to Dr. Jennifer Wilson, Dr. Raja Abboud, Dr. Peter Paré, Dr. Najib Ayas, Dr. Mark Fitzgerald, Dr. John Fleetham, Dr. John Granton, and Dr. John Marshall. We also acknowledge Dr. Abdulaziz Alsaif, Dr. Turki Altassan, and Dr. Majdi Idris. A special thanks to Bernice Robillard.

Contents

Chapter 1
Spirometry

Spirometry is the most essential part of any pulmonary function study and provides the most information. In spirometry, a machine called a spirometer is used to measure certain lung volumes, called dynamic lung volumes. The two most important dynamic lung volumes measured are the forced vital capacity (FVC) and the forced expiratory volume in the 1st second (FEV_1). This section deals with the definitions of these and other terms.

DEFINITIONS[1, 2]

Forced Vital Capacity

- Is the volume of air in liters that can be forcefully and maximally exhaled after a maximal inspiration. FVC is unique and reproducible for a given subject.
- The *slow vital capacity (SVC)* – also called the *vital capacity (VC)* – is similar to the FVC, but the exhalation is slow rather than being as rapid as possible as in the FVC. In a normal subject, the SVC usually equals the FVC,[3] while in patients with an obstructive lung disorder (see Table 1.1 for definition), the SVC is usually larger than the FVC. The reason for this is that, in obstructive lung disorders, the airways tend to collapse and close prematurely because of the increased positive intrathoracic pressure during a forceful expiration. This increased pressure leads to air trapping. Accordingly, a significantly higher SVC compared with FVC suggests air-trapping; Figure 1.1.
- The *inspiratory vital capacity (IVC)* is the VC measured during inspiration rather than expiration. The IVC should equal the expiratory VC. If it does not, poor effort or an air leak could be

1

Ali Altalag et al., *Pulmonary Function Tests in Clinical Practice*,
DOI: 10.1007/978-1-84882-231-3_1,
© Springer-Verlag London Limited 2009

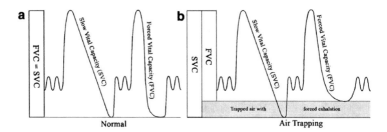

FIGURE 1.1. FVC and SVC are compared with each other in a normal subject (**a**) and in a patient with an obstructive disorder (**b**). In case of airway obstruction, SVC is larger than FVC, indicating air trapping.

responsible. IVC may be larger than the expiratory VC in patients with significant airway obstruction, as in this case the increased negative intrathoracic pressure opens the airways facilitating inspiration, as opposed to the narrowing of airways during exhalation as the intrathoracic pressure becomes positive.[4, 5] Narrowed airways reduce airflow and hence the amount of exhaled air.

Forced Expiratory Volume in the 1st Second

- Is the volume of air in liters that can be forcefully and maximally exhaled in the 1st second after a maximal inspiration. In other words, it is the volume of air that is exhaled in the 1st second of the FVC, and it normally represents ~80% of the FVC.
- FEV_6 is similarly defined as the volume of air exhaled in the first 6 s of the FVC and its only significance is that it can sometimes substitute the FVC in patients who fail to exhale completely.[6]

FEV_1/FVC Ratio

- This ratio is used to differentiate obstructive from restrictive lung disorders; see Table 1.1 for definitions. In obstructive disorders, FEV_1 drops much more significantly than FVC and the ratio will be low, while in restrictive disorders, the ratio is either normal or even increased as the drop in FVC is either proportional to or more marked than the drop in FEV_1.
- Normally, the FEV_1/FVC ratio is greater than 0.7, but it decreases (to values <0.7) with normal aging.[7] In children, however, it is higher and can reach as high as 0.9.[8] The changes in the elderly probably reflect the decrease in elastic recoil of the lungs that occurs with aging.

TABLE 1.1. Definitions of obstructive and restrictive disorders

Obstructive disorders

Are characterized by diffuse airway narrowing secondary to different
    mechanisms [immune related, e.g., bronchial asthma, or environmental,
    e.g., chronic obstructive pulmonary disease (COPD)]

Restrictive disorders

Are a group of disorders characterized by abnormal reduction of the lung
    volumes, either because of alteration in the lung parenchyma or
    because of a disease of the pleura, chest wall or due to muscle weakness

The Instantaneous Forced Expiratory Flow (FEF_{25}, FEF_{50}, FEF_{75}) and the Maximum Mid-Expiratory Flow (MMEF or FEF_{25-75})

- The instantaneous forced expiratory flow (FEF) represents the
  flow of the exhaled air measured (in liters per second) at different points of the FVC, namely at 25, 50, and 75% of the FVC.
  They are abbreviated as FEF_{25}, FEF_{50}, and FEF_{75}, respectively;
  Figure 1.2b. The maximum mid-expiratory flow (MMEF) or
  FEF_{25-75}, however, is the average flow during the middle half
  of the FVC (25–75% of FVC); see Figure 1.2c. These variables
  represent the effort-independent part of the FVC.[9] Collectively,
  they are considered more sensitive (but non-specific) in detecting early airway obstruction, which tends to take place at lower
  lung volumes.[10,11] Their usefulness is limited, however, because
  of the wide range of normal values.[10]

Peak Expiratory Flow

- Is the maximum flow (in liters per second) of air during a forceful exhalation. Normally, it takes place immediately after the
  start of the exhalation and it is effort-dependent. PEF drops with
  a poor initial effort and in obstructive and, to a lesser extent,
  restrictive disorders. PEF measured in the laboratory is similar
  to the peak expiratory flow (PEF) rate (in liters per minute)
  that is measured routinely at the bedside to monitor asthmatic
  patients.

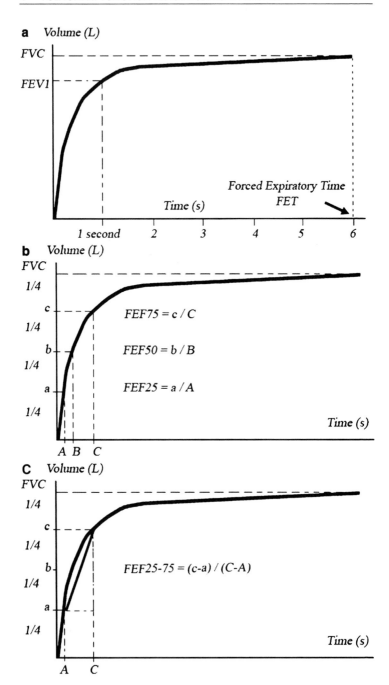

SPIROMETRIC CURVES

The Volume–Time Curve (The Spirogram)

- Is simply the FVC plotted as volume in liters against time in seconds; Figure 1.2a.
- You can extract from this curve both the FVC and FEV_1. FEV_1/FVC ratio can be estimated by looking at where the FEV_1 stands in relation to the FVC in the volume axis; Figure 1.2a. In addition, the curve's shape helps in determining that ratio: a decreased ratio will necessarily make the curve look flatter and less steep than normal; see Figure 1.16. The FEFs (FEF_{25}, FEF_{50}, FEF_{75}) and MMEF (FEF_{25-75}) can also be roughly estimated from the curve as shown in Figure 1.2b, c.
- This curve also provides an idea about the quality of the spirometry, as it shows the duration of the exhalation [the forced expiratory time (FET)], which needs to be at least 6 s for the study to be clinically reliable. Quality control will be explained in more detail later in this chapter.
- If a postbronchodilator study is done, as in case of suspected bronchial asthma, then there will be two discrete curves. One curve will represent the initial (prebronchodilator) study whereas the second will represent the postbronchodilator study. Looking at how the two curves compare to each other gives an idea about the degree of the response to bronchodilator therapy, if any; Figure 1.16.

FIGURE 1.2. The volume–time curve (spirogram). The following data can be acquired: (**a**) FVC is the highest point in the curve; FEV_1 is plotted in the volume axis opposite to the point in the curve corresponding to 1 s; duration of the study (the forced expiratory time or FET) can be determined from the time axis, 6 s in this curve. (**b**) $FEF_{25,50,75}$ can be roughly determined by dividing the volume axis into four quarters and determining the corresponding time for each quarter from the time axis. Dividing the volumes (a, b, and c) by the corresponding time (A, B, and C) gives the value of each FEF (FEF_{25}, FEF_{50}, FEF_{75}, respectively). Note that this method represents a rough determination of FEFs, as FEFs are actually measured instantaneously by the spirometer and not calculated. (**c**) FEF_{25-75} can be roughly determined by dividing the volume during the middle half of the FVC (c–a) by the corresponding time (C–A). FEF_{25-75} represents the slope of the curve at those two points.

The Expiratory Flow–Volume Curve (FV Curve)

- Is determined by plotting FVC as flow (in liters per second) against volume (in liters); Figure 1.3.* This curve is more informative and easier to interpret, as different diseases produce distinct curve shapes.

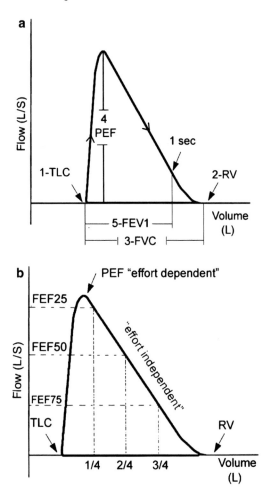

---

* The flow can be measured directly by a pneumotachograph. The volume is obtained by integration of the flow signal. Alternatively, a volume sensing device (spirometer) measures volume and the flow is derived by differentiating the volume signal. Either method allows expression of the flow–volume curve.

- The curve starts at full inspiration (at the *total lung capacity or TLC*: the total amount of air in the lungs at maximal inhalation; Figure 1.3a) with 0 flow (just before the patient starts exhaling), then the flow or speed of the exhaled air increases exponentially and rapidly reaches its maximum, which is the PEF. The curve then starts sloping down in an almost linear way until just before reaching the volume axis when it curves less steeply giving a small upward concavity. The curve then ends in that way at the *residual volume or RV* (the amount of air that remains in the lungs after a maximal exhalation) by touching the volume axis, i.e., a flow of 0 (or within 0.1 L/s)[8] when no more air can be exhaled; Figure 1.3a.
- As you notice, there is no time axis in this curve, and the only way to determine the FEV_1 is by the reading device making a 1st second mark on the curve, which is normally located at ~ 80% of the FVC. See Figure 1.3a.
- Other data can be extracted from this curve including $FEF_{25, 50, 75}$ as shown in Figure 1.3b. FEF_{25-75} cannot be determined from this curve.
- In summary, every part of the curve represents something; Figure 1.3:
  - The leftmost end of the curve represents TLC.
  - The curve's rightmost end represents RV.
  - Its width represents FVC.
  - Its height represents PEF.
  - The distance from TLC to the 1-s mark represents FEV_1.
  - The descending slope reflects the FEFs.
- Remember that we cannot measure RV and hence TLC with spirometry alone, because we cannot measure the air remaining in the lung after a full exhalation with this method. Methods that can measure RV are discussed in the next chapter.
- The morphology of the curve is as important as the other values. It provides information about the quality of the study as well as being able to recognize certain disease states from its shape. These will be explained in detail later in this chapter.

FIGURE 1.3. (**a**) The flow–volume curve: the following data can be extracted: (1) TLC is represented by the leftmost end of the curve (cannot be measured by spirometry); (2) RV is represented by the rightmost end of the curve (cannot be measured by spirometry); (3) FVC is represented by the width of the curve; (4) PEF is represented by the height of the curve; (5) FEV_1 is the distance from TLC to the 1st second mark. (**b**) The flow–volume curve demonstrating the effort-dependent and the effort-independent parts. Instantaneous FEFs are directly determined from the curve by dividing the FVC into four quarters and getting the corresponding flow for the first, second, and third quarters representing $FEF_{25,50,75}$, respectively as shown. The FEFs represent the slope of the FV curve.

- Two curves are often shown in different colors (blue and red) to depict pre- and postbronchodilator studies, respectively, if a postbronchodilator study was done; Figure 1.15b.

The Maximal Flow–Volume Loop

- Combining the expiratory flow–volume curve, discussed earlier, with the inspiratory curve (that measures the IVC) produces the maximal flow–volume loop, with the expiratory curve forming the upper and the inspiratory curve forming the lower parts of that loop; see Figure 1.4.
- This loop is even more informative than the expiratory flow–volume curve alone, as it also provides information about the inspiratory portion of the breathing cycle. For example, extrathoracic upper airway obstruction, which occurs during inspiration, can now be detected.
- This loop commonly includes a tidal flow–volume loop too, shown in the center of the maximal flow–volume loop as a small circle; Figure 1.4. This loop represents quiet breathing. Additional useful data can be acquired from this tidal loop when compared with the maximal flow–volume loop. These useful data include the *expiratory reserve volume (ERV)* and the *inspiratory capacity (IC)*; Figure 1.4b – see next chapter for definitions. The values of ERV and IC estimated from this curve might be slightly different from the lung volume study measurements, where the SVC is measured instead of the FVC as these (FVC and SVC) can be different in some disorders such as obstructive disorders, as was discussed earlier. More details about these measurements will be discussed in the following chapter.

TECHNIQUE OF SPIROMETRY[1]

- The spirometer – the machine used to record spirometry – has to be calibrated every morning to ensure that it records accurate values before it is used. The temperature and barometric pressure are entered into the spirometer every morning, as variation in these measures does affect the final results[†].[12–14]
- The patient must be clinically stable, should sit straight, with head erect, nose clip in place, and holding the mouthpiece tightly between the lips. Initially, he or she should breathe in and

---

[†]As air in the lungs is at BTPS (body temperature pressure standard) but collected at ATPS (ambient temperature pressure standard), a correction factor has to be applied to obtain the BTPS volumes as these are the reported volumes.

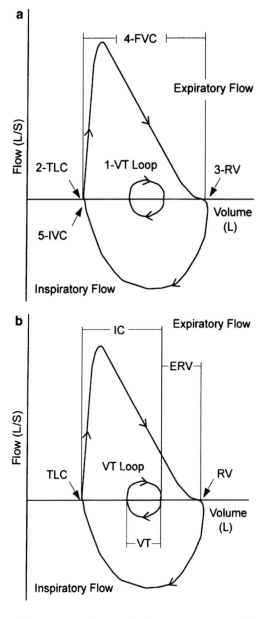

FIGURE 1.4. (**a**) Represents the steps in data measurement during spirometry. (**b**) Demonstrates the ERV and IC in relation to the tidal flow–volume loop (V_T stands for tidal volume).

out at the tidal volume (V_T: normal quiet breathing) to record the tidal flow–volume loop; Figure 1.4a, No. 1. Then, when the patient is ready, the technician instructs him/her to inhale maximally to TLC (Figure 1.4a, No. 2), and then exhale as fast and as completely as possible to record the FVC (Figure 1.4a, No. 4). The point at which no more air can be exhaled is the RV (Figure 1.4a, No. 3). The patient is then instructed to inhale fully to TLC again in order to record the IVC (Figure 1.4a, No. 5). This test is then repeated to ensure reproducibility in order to meet quality control criteria (American Thoracic Society or ATS criteria); see next section.

- If a bronchodilator study is needed, then the test is repeated in the same way 10 min after giving the patient a short-acting β_2 agonist (usually 2–4 puffs of salbutamol through a spacer chamber). The ATS criteria should be met in the postbronchodilator study too.
- The spirometer will produce the volume as absolute numbers and as curves.
- The technician should make a note to the interpreting doctor of any technical difficulty that may have influenced the quality of the study. Technician's comments are important as are the ATS criteria in the final report.

THE ATS GUIDELINES[1,2]

The ATS criteria are easy to remember. They include both acceptability and reproducibility criteria. This means that each individual study should meet certain criteria to be accepted, and the accepted studies should not vary more than predefined limits to ensure reproducibility. If either of the criteria are not met, then the study is rejected as it may give a false impression of either normal or abnormal lung function. Of course, bedside tests or field testing, e.g., in the emergency department, do not, in many instances, meet the ATS criteria that are required for measures in an accredited laboratory.

Acceptability[1,2]

The ATS mandates three acceptable maneuvers. The number of trials that can be performed on an individual should not exceed 8. An acceptable trial should have a good start, a good end, and absence of artifacts.

1. Good start of the test:
   - If the study needs back extrapolation, the extrapolation volume should not exceed 5% of FVC or 150 ml, whichever is larger. See Figure 1.5.[1,2,15–19]

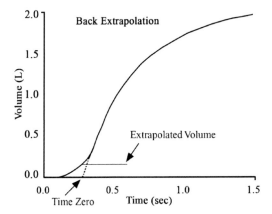

FIGURE 1.5. Extrapolation volume of 150 ml or 5% of FVC (whichever is larger) (with permission from American Thoracic Society[2]).

Note: Back extrapolation applies to the VT curve and means that if the start of the test is not optimal, correction can be made by shifting the time axis forward, provided that the extrapolation volume is within either one of the limits mentioned earlier. To simplify this, consider that a patient's FVC is 2 L and the study requires a back extrapolation correction, and 5% of the FVC (2 L) is 100 ml. Because 150 ml is larger than 5% of the patient's FVC (100 ml), 150 ml should be used as the upper limit of extrapolated volume. Then, if the measured extrapolated volume is greater than 150 ml, the result cannot be accepted.

Note: A good start of the study can be identified qualitatively on the FV curve as a rapid rise of flow to PEF from the baseline (0 point), with the PEF being sharp and rounded. The FEV_1 can be over- or underestimated with submaximal effort, which may mimic lung disorders such as those due to airway obstruction or lung restriction; see later.[2,20]

2. Smooth flow–volume (FV) curve, free of artifacts[1,2]:

These artifacts will show in both volume–time (VT) and FV curves but will be more pronounced in the FV curve. These artifacts include the following:

(a) *Cough during the 1st second of exhalation* may significantly affect FEV_1. The FV curve is sensitive in detecting this artifact; Figure 1.6. Coughing after the 1st second is less likely to make a significant difference in the FVC and so it is accepted provided that it does not distort the shape of the FV curve (judged by the technician).[1]

(b) Variable effort; Figure 1.7.
(c) Glottis closure; Figure 1.8.
(d) Early termination of effort.

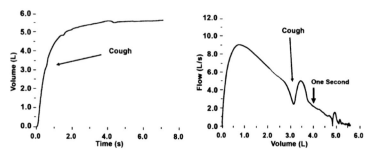

FIGURE 1.6. Cough in the 1st second. It is much clearer in the FV curve than in the VT curve as indicated by the *arrows* (with permission from American Thoracic Society[2]).

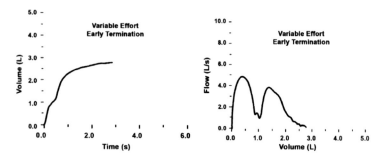

FIGURE 1.7. Variable effort: any study with a variable effort is rejected (with permission from American Thoracic Society[2]).

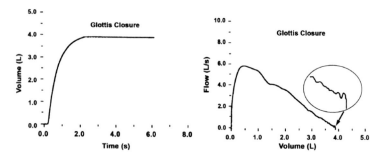

FIGURE 1.8. Glottis closure (with permission from American Thoracic Society[2]).

(e) Obstructed mouthpiece, by applying the tongue through the mouthpiece or biting it with the teeth.

(f) *Air leak*[1,2,16,21]:
- The air leak source could be due to loose tube connections or, more commonly, because the patient weakly applies lips around the mouthpiece. Air leak can be detected from the FV loop; Figure 1.11e.

3. Good end of the test (demonstrated in the VT curve):

(a) Plateau of VT curve of at least 1 s, i.e., volume is not changing much with time indicating that the patient is approaching the residual volume (RV).[1,2]

OR

(b) Reasonable duration of effort (FET)[1,2]:
- Six seconds is the minimum accepted duration (3 s for children[1]).
- Ten seconds is the optimal.[22]
- FET of >15 s is unlikely to change the clinical decision and may result in the patient's exhaustion.[1] Patients with obstructive disorders can exhale for more than 40 s before reaching their RV, i.e., before reaching a plateau in the VT curve; Figure 1.9. Normal individuals, however, can empty their lung (i.e., reach a plateau) within 4 s.

OR

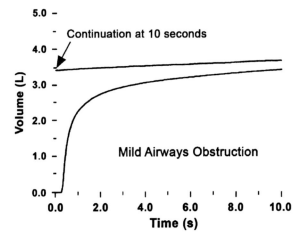

FIGURE 1.9. Mild airway obstruction, with prolonged duration of exhalation (20 s). Notice that, when the curve exceeds the limit of the time axis, the continuation of the curve will be plotted from the beginning of the time axis (with permission from American Thoracic Society[2]).

(c) The patient cannot or should not continue to exhale.[1,2]

Note: A good end of the study can be shown in the FV curve as an upward concavity at the end of the curve. A downward concavity, however, indicates that the patient either stopped exhaling (prematurely) or started inhaling before reaching the RV; Figure 1.10. This poor technique may result in underestimation of the FVC.[10]

- Figure 1.11 shows the morphology of FV curve in acceptable and unacceptable maneuvers.

Reproducibility[1,2]

- After obtaining three acceptable maneuvers, the following reproducibility criteria should be applied:
  - The two largest values of FVC must be within 150 ml of each other.
  - The two largest values of FEV_1 must be within 150 ml of each other.
- If the studies are not reproducible, then the studies should be repeated until the ATS criteria are met or a total of eight trials are completed or the patient either cannot or should not continue testing.[1,2]

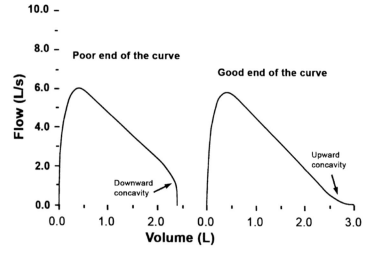

FIGURE 1.10. Poor end in comparison to good end (small upward concavity) of FV curve. A poor end (downward concavity) indicates premature termination of exhalation (before 0 flow).

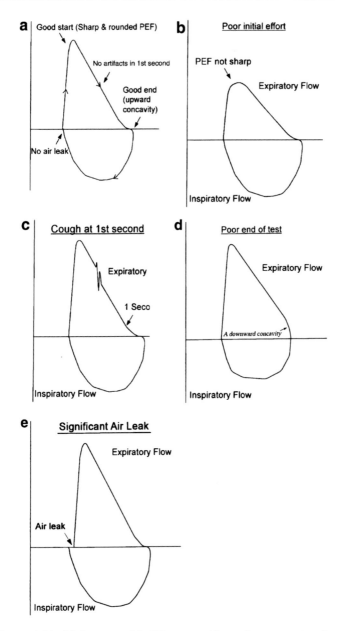

FIGURE 1.11. (a) An acceptable FV curve, with good start, good end, and free from artifacts. (b) Shows a poor start. (c) Shows a cough in the 1st second. (d) Shows a poor end. (e) Shows air leak.

- The final values should be chosen based on the following[1,2]:
  - FEV$_1$ and FVC should be reported as the highest values from any acceptable/reproducible trial (not necessarily from the same trial).
  - The other flow parameters should be taken from the best test curve (which is the curve with the highest sum of FVC + FEV$_1$).
  - If reproducibility cannot be achieved after eight trials, the best test curve (the highest acceptable trial) should be reported. The technician should comment on this deviation from protocol so that the interpreting physician understands that the results may not be accurate.
- Finally, acceptable trials are not necessarily reproducible, because the patient may not produce maximum effort in all trials. Figures 1.12 and 1.13 give some useful examples.[2]

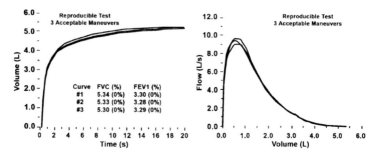

FIGURE 1.12. Acceptable and reproducible trials (with permission from American Thoracic Society[2]).

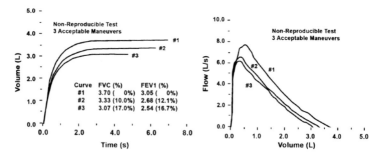

FIGURE 1.13. Acceptable but not reproducible trials (With permission from: American Thoracic Society[2]).

TABLE 1.2. Features of the ideal FV and VT curves

The ideal FV curve should have the following features; Figure 1.11a:
    Good start with sharp and rounded PEF
    Smooth continuous decline free from artifacts
    Good end with a small upward concavity at or near the 0 flow

The ideal VT curve should either have a plateau for 1 s *or* show an effort of at least 6 s

- Now, by looking at any FV curve, you should be able to tell whether or not it reflects an acceptable study. Table 1.2 summarizes the features of the ideal FV and VT curves. Keep in mind that the lack of any of these features may indicate a lung disorder rather than a poor study.

REFERENCE VALUES[10,23–27]

- The reference values for the PFT have a wide range of normal as the lung size varies considerably in the normal subjects. These values depend on certain variables:
  - Sex (Men have bigger lungs than women.)
  - Age (The spirometric values drop with age.)
  - Height (Tall people have bigger lungs. If it is difficult to measure the height, as in kyphoscoliosis, then the arm span can be measured instead.[14,28])
  - A fourth important variable is race (Caucasians have bigger lungs than Africans and Asians), related to differing body proportions (legs to torso)
- Spirometric measurements from a group of healthy subjects with a given sex, age, height, and race usually exhibit a normal distribution curve; Figure 1.14. The 5th percentile (1.65 standard deviations) is, then, used to define the lower limit of the reference range for that given sex, age, height, and race; Figure 1.14.[10,27]
- The available reference values apply only to Caucasians on whom the original studies were performed. Blacks are well studied too, and they generally have lower predicted values than the Caucasians, although they are usually taller, because blacks have higher leg length to torso length ratios, i.e., smaller lungs. So, while interpreting the lung functions of a black American, you need to make race-specific corrections to the standard predicted values; Table 1.3.[10,27]
- Asians also have lower values than the standard predicted values. An adjustment factor of 0.94 is recommended for Asian Americans.[29,30]

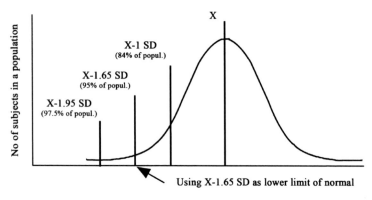

Figure 1.14. The predicted values for a group of normal subjects at a given height, age, and sex form a normal distribution curve. Applying 1.65 standard deviations (the 5th percentile) to define the lower limit of normal will include 95% of that population.

TABLE 1.3. Correction factors for the PFT of Black Americans

Variable	Correction factor
FEV_1, FVC, TLC	0.88
RV, DL_{CO}	0.93
FEV_1/FVC ratio	1 (i.e., no correction needed)

Blacks have smaller lungs than Caucasians and their lung function values need to be adjusted by multiplying these correction factors by the reference values acquired from Caucasian studies.[10,27]

• The standard normal values roughly range from 80 to 120% of the predicted values that are derived from Caucasian studies.[‡] When you interpret a PFT, you should always look at the patient's results as percentage of the predicted values for that particular patient (written in the report as % pred.). If the patient is normal, then his/her values should roughly lie within 80–120% of predicted values.[*]

[‡] Using a fixed value of the lower limit of normal (80%) may be accepted in children but may lead to some errors in adults.[27]

[*] As can be seen in figure 1.14 the 95% confidence limit may be used for normality as well. Values outside this range are then below the limit of normal (LLN). Many software programs for lung function testing can display the LLN and interpreting physicians may use this to determine normality. The predicted values used (reference equations) should be representative of the population being tested.

- The absolute value for each variable has some significance. As an example, FVC equals roughly 5 L in an average young adult. This number could vary significantly among normal individuals, but if somebody tells you that your patient's FVC is 1 L, you will know that this is far below the expected for an average young adult and will warrant some attention.

GRADING OF SEVERITY

- Different variables and values were used to grade severity of different pulmonary disorders[10,27,31–33];
- Recently, FEV_1 has been selected to grade severity of any spirometric abnormality (obstructive, restrictive, or mixed); Table 1.4.[10] The traditional way of grading severity of obstructive and restrictive disorders involve the following:
  - In obstructive disorders, the FEV_1/FVC ratio should be <0.7, and the value of FEV_1 is used to determine severity[27]; Table 1.4.
  - In restrictive disorders, however, FEV_1/FVC ratio is normal and the TLC is less than 80% predicted. The ATS suggested using the TLC to grade the severity of restrictive disorders, which cannot be measured in simple spirometry.[27] Where only spirometry is available, FVC may be used to make that grading.[27] The TLC, however, should be known before confidently diagnosing a restrictive disorder[27,34,35]; Table 1.4.

BRONCHODILATOR RESPONSE

- Bronchodilators can be used in selected patients following the initial spirometry. Response to bronchodilators suggests asthma, but other obstructive lung disorders can respond to bronchodilators as well, i.e., chronic obstructive pulmonary disease (COPD). Normal subjects can also respond to bronchodilators by as much as 8% increase in FVC and FEV_1, but this change is not considered significant.[36,37] The bronchodilator of choice is salbutamol delivered by metered dose inhaler (MDI), through a spacer.[§38–45]
- For the test to be accurate, patients are advised to stop taking any short-acting β_2 agonists or anticholinergic agents within 4 h of testing.[1] Long-acting β_2 agonists (like formoterol and salmeterol) and oral aminophylline should be stopped at least 12 h before the test.[1] Smoking should be avoided for ≥1 h prior to testing

---

§A spacer is an attachment to the MDI, which optimizes the delivery of salbutamol.

TABLE 1.4. Methods of grading the severity of obstructive and restrictive disorders

(A) Grading of severity of any spirometric abnormality based on FEV_1[10]	
After determining the pattern to be obstructive, restrictive, or mixed, FEV_1 is used to grade severity:	
Mild	$FEV_1 > 70$ (% pred.)
Moderate	60–69
Moderately Severe	50–59
Severe	35–49
Very severe	<35

(B) Traditional method of grading the severity of obstructive and restrictive disorders*[,27]	
• Obstructive disorder (based on FEV_1) – Ratio < 0.7	
May be a physiologic variant	$FEV_1 \geq 100$ (% pred.)
Mild	70–100
Moderate	60–69
Moderately severe	50–59
Severe	35–49
Very severe	<35
• Restrictive disorder (based on TLC, preferred)	
Mild	TLC > 70 (% pred.)
Moderate	60–69
Severe	<60
• Restrictive disorder (based on FVC, in case no lung volume study is available)	
Mild	FVC > 70 (% pred.)
Moderate	60–69
Moderately severe	50–59
Severe	35–49
Very severe	<35

*This is a widely used grading system but different organizations use different systems of grading.

and throughout the procedure.[1,14] Caffeine-containing substances should be avoided the day of testing. Inhaled or systemic steroids do not interfere with the test results, and so, they do not need to be stopped.[8] The technicians' comment should indicate if a patient has just had a bronchodilator prior to the study.

- The definition of a significant response to bronchodilators according to ATS & ERS (European Respiratory Society) is increase in FEV_1 or FVC by >12% and >200 ml in the postbronchodilator study.[¶][10,46]

COMPONENTS OF SPIROMETRY

- Table 1.5 summarizes the causes of abnormal spirometric components. In any spirometry report, you may see multiple other parameters that are not discussed here and have little or even no clinical usefulness. For the purpose of completeness, these components are also shown in this table.
- Table 1.6 summarizes the effects of different lung disorders on every component of spirometry.

SPIROMETRIC PATTERN OF COMMON DISORDERS

In this section, we will discuss the PFT pattern of some common disorders.

Obstructive Disorders

- The two major obstructive disorders are bronchial asthma and COPD; Table 1.7. The key to the diagnosis of these disorders is the drop in FEV_1/FVC ratio.[10] FEV_1 may be reduced too and is used to define the severity of obstruction; see Table 1.4. FVC may be reduced in obstructive disorders but usually not to the same degree as FEV_1.
- The features of obstructive disorders are summarized in Table 1.6.
- The flow–volume curve can be used alone to confidently make the diagnosis of obstructive disorders, as it has a distinct shape in such disorders; Figure 1.15. These features include the following:
  - The height of the curve (PEF) is much less than predicted.
  - The descending limb is concave (scooped), with the outward concavity being more pronounced with more severe obstruction. The slope of the descending limb that represents MMEF and FEFs is reduced due to airflow limitation at low lung volumes.

¶Increments of as high as 8% or 150 ml in FEV_1 or FVC are likely to be within the variability of the measurement.[36,56]

TABLE 1.5. Causes of abnormal spirometric components

FVC
Increased in acromegaly[8]
Decreased in restrictive disorders (most important) and obstructive disorders; Table 1.6

FEV_1
Decreased in obstructive and, to a lesser extent, restrictive disorders

FEV_1/FVC ratio
Increased in interstitial lung diseases (ILD) such as pulmonary fibrosis (because of increased elastic recoil that results in a relatively preserved FEV_1)
Decreased in obstructive disorders (asthma and COPD)

PEF
May be increased in pulmonary fibrosis (because of increased elastic recoil)
Decreased in the following:
Obstructive disorders (COPD, asthma)
Intrathoracic or fixed upper airway obstruction[10,46,47] (associated with flattening of the expiratory curve of the flow–volume loop)
Restrictive disorders other than pulmonary fibrosis

$FEF_{(25, 50, 75, 25-75)}$
Decreased in obstructive and restrictive disorders
Decreased also in variable extrathoracic or fixed upper airway obstruction
Reduction in FEF_{75} and/or FEF_{25-75} may be the earliest sign of airflow obstruction in small airways.[10,48-50] This sign, however, is not specific for small airway disease.[11]

FET (forced expiratory time)
May be increased in obstructive disorders

PIF (peak inspiratory flow)
Decreased in variable extrathoracic or fixed upper airway obstruction

FIF_{50} (forced inspiratory flow at 50% of FIVC)
Decreased in variable extrathoracic or fixed upper airway obstruction

FIVC (forced inspiratory vital capacity)
Its main use is to check for the quality of the study (for air leak)

FIF_{50}/FEF_{50}
Increased in variable intrathoracic upper airway obstruction (>1)[10]
Decreased in variable extrathoracic upper airway obstruction (<1), see also Table 1.9.[10]

TABLE 1.6. Features of obstructive and restrictive disorders

Features of obstructive disorders
  Diagnostic features: $\downarrow$ FEV_1/FVC ratio
  Other features:
    $\downarrow$ FEV_1
    $\downarrow$ FVC (can be normal)
    $\downarrow$ FEFs and MMEF (FEF_{25}, $FEF_{50,}$ FEF_{75}, FEF_{25-75})
    $\downarrow$ PEF
    $\downarrow$ FET
    Significant bronchodilator response
    Scooped (concave) descending limb of FV curve

Features of restrictive disorders
  Most important features: $\downarrow$ FVC and normal or $\uparrow$ FEV_1/FVC ratio
  Other features:
    $\downarrow$ FEV_1 (proportional to FVC), but it can be normal
    $\downarrow$ MMEF
    PEF: normal, increased, or decreased
    Steep descending limb of FV curve

TABLE 1.7. Causes of obstructive and restrictive disorders

Causes of obstructive disorders
  Bronchial asthma (usually responsive to bronchodilators)
  COPD

Causes of restrictive disorders
  Parenchymal disease as pulmonary fibrosis and other interstitial lung
    diseases (ILD)
  Pleural disease as pleural fibrosis (uncommon)
  Chest wall restriction:
    Musculoskeletal disorders (MSD), e.g. severe kyphoscoliosis
    Neuromuscular disorders (NMD), e.g. muscular dystrophy, amyotrophic
      lateral sclerosis (ALS), old poliomyelitis, paralyzed diaphragm;
      see Table 5.1 for more detail.
    Diaphragmatic distention (pregnancy, ascites, obesity)
    Obesity (restricting chest wall movement)
  Loss of air spaces:
    Resection (lobectomy, pneumonectomy)
    Atelectasis
    Tumors (filling or compressing alveolar spaces)
    Pulmonary edema (alveolar spaces become filled with fluid)
    Pleural cavity disease (pleural effusion, extensive cardiomegaly, large
      pleural tumor)

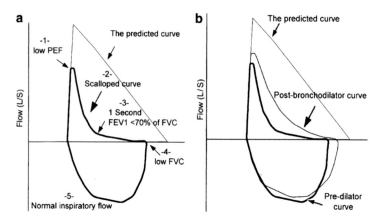

FIGURE 1.15. Obstructive disorders (FV curve): (**a**) The FV curve looks technically acceptable, with good start and end, and absence of artifacts in the 1st second. There are five features that make the diagnosis of a significant airway obstruction definite, based on this curve alone. 1 – Decreased PEF when compared to the predicted curve. 2 – Scooping of the curve after PEF, indicating airflow limitation. 3 – The 1st second mark is almost in the middle of the curve indicating that the FEV_1 and FEV_1/FVC ratio are significantly decreased. 4 – FVC is decreased when compared to the predicted curve. 5 – The inspiratory component of the curve is normal, excluding a central airway obstruction. (**b**) There is a clear response to bronchodilators indicating reversibility and supporting the diagnosis of an obstructive disorder, most likely bronchial asthma.

- Decreased FEV_1 and FEV_1/FVC ratio are easily noted by identifying the 1st second mark (FEV_1) and where it lies in relation to the FVC.
- The width of the curve (FVC) as seen in the volume axis may be decreased compared with that of the predicted curve.
- A postbronchodilator study, represented by the red curve, demonstrates an improvement in all of the aforementioned variables [PEF, the curve's outward concavity (FEF), FEV_1, FEV_1/FVC ratio, and FVC]; Figure 1.15b. These improvements strongly suggest a specific obstructive disorder, namely asthma. Lack of bronchodilator response does not exclude bronchial asthma as responsiveness can vary over time. Similarly many patients with COPD can show reversibility. Reversibility in the correct clinical context (i.e. young non-smoker) supports the diagnosis of asthma.
- The VT curve similarly has its distinct features of obstructive disorders; Figure 1.16.

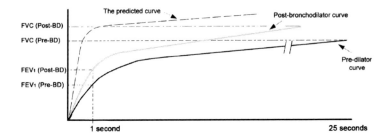

FIGURE 1.16. Feature of obstructive disorders in VT curve: 1 – The *black curve* (prebronchodilator study) is less steep compared with the *dashed curve* (the predicted). 2 – FEV$_1$ and the FEV$_1$/FVC ratio are decreased in the *black curve*. 3 – The FVC is also decreased. 4 – A prolonged FET (length of the curve) suggests airway obstruction. 5 – MMEF is also decreased, indicated by the slope of the curve. 6 – The curve morphology improves following bronchodilator therapy (the *gray curve*), with subsequent improvement of FEV$_1$, FVC, and FEV$_1$/FVC ratio.

- Special Conditions
  - In mild (or early) airway obstruction, the classic reduction in FEV$_1$ and FEV$_1$/FVC ratio may not be seen. The morphology of the FV curve can give a clue, as the distal upward concavity may show to be more pronounced and prolonged; Figure 1.17.[48–50] Another clue is the prolonged FET evident in the VT curve; Figure 1.17. However, the clinical significance of these mild changes is unknown.
  - In emphysema and because of loss of supportive tissues, the airways tend to collapse significantly at low lung volumes, giving a characteristic "dog-leg" appearance in FV curve; Figure 1.18.[9]

Restrictive Disorders

- In restrictive disorders, such as pulmonary fibrosis, the key to the diagnosis is the drop in FVC, as the volume of the air spaces is significantly lower than normal. The lung elasticity increases and the lungs retract. The FEV$_1$/FVC ratio has to be preserved or increased, however.[10] To make a confident diagnosis of a restrictive disorder, the TLC should be measured and should be low.[27,34,35] So, based on spirometry alone, the earlier features are reported as suggestive (not diagnostic) of a restrictive disorder. Remember that normal FVC or VC excludes lung restriction.[34,35]
- Table 1.6 summarizes the features of a restrictive disorder in spirometry and Table 1.7 summarizes the etiology.

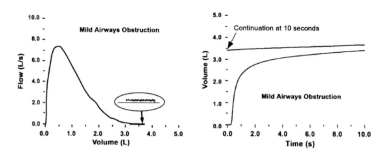

FIGURE 1.17. Mild airway obstruction (with permission from American Thoracic Society[2]).

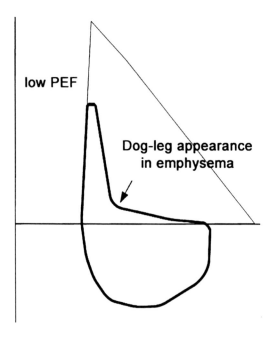

FIGURE 1.18. *Dog-leg* appearance typical of emphysema.

- FV curve features of restrictive disorders are described as follows:
  - For parenchymal lung disease (e.g., pulmonary fibrosis); Figure 1.19a:
    (a) The PEF can be normal or high because of the increased elastic recoil that increases the initial flow of exhaled air.

However, PEF may be low as the disease progresses due to the reduced volumes exhaled, i.e., fewer liters per second.

(b) The width of the curve (FVC) is decreased and the 1st second mark (FEV_1) on the descending limb of the curve is close to the residual volume indicating a normal or high FEV_1/FVC ratio.

(c) The slope of the descending limb of the curve is steeper than usual due to high lung recoil or elastance (i.e., low MMEF). The reduction in MMEF, in this case, does not indicate air-flow obstruction and is related to the reduced volumes.

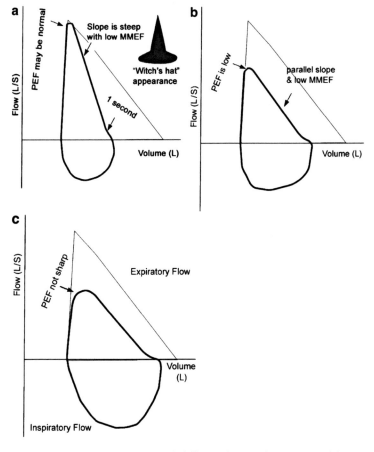

FIGURE 1.19. FV curve features of different forms of restriction: (**a**) ILD with witch's hat appearance; (**b**) chest wall restriction (excluding NMD); (**c**) NMD (or poor effort study) producing a convex curve.

(d) The steep descending limb and the narrow width of the FV curve together with the relatively preserved PEF may produce a distinct shape of the curve typical for parenchymal lung fibrosis referred to as the *witch's hat appearance*.
- For chest wall restriction (including musculoskeletal disorders, diaphragmatic distention, and obesity); Figure 1.19b:
  (a) PEF is decreased as the elastic recoil of the lung is not increased here.
  (b) The slope of the curve is parallel to the predicted curve, making the whole curve looking like the predicted curve but smaller. The MMEF is similarly decreased.
- For neuromuscular disorders (this pattern is also seen in poor effort study); Figure 1.19c:
  (a) The PEF is low and not sharp (the curve is convex in shape).
  (b) The MMEF is low.
- The volume–time (VT) curve will maintain the normal morphology but will be smaller than the predicted curve in restrictive disorders.

Upper Airway Obstruction[51–55]

The morphology of the flow–volume curve is very useful in identifying upper airway disorders. However, these disorders must be advanced to allow detection by this technique. There are three types of upper airway obstruction recognizable in the FV curve:

1. *Variable extrathoracic obstruction* (above the level of sternal notch)
   (a) The word variable means that the obstruction comes and goes during a maximum inspiratory or expiratory effort, unlike a fixed obstruction that never changes with forced efforts. In variable extrathoracic obstruction, airway obstruction takes place during inspiration. This is because the pressure inside the airways (larynx, pharynx, extrathoracic portion of trachea) is relatively negative during inspiration compared with the pressure outside the airways (atmospheric pressure, P_{atm}) and hence flow is reduced (flattened curve) during the inspiratory limb of the FV curve; Figure 1.20a. The obstruction has to be mobile or dynamic to follow this pattern. Patients with such lesions develop stridor, i.e., a wheezy sound during inspiration.
2. *Variable intrathoracic obstruction* (below the sternal notch)
   (a) In this case, the obstruction will be more pronounced during expiration. The central intrathoracic airways (intrathoracic trachea and main bronchi) narrow when they are compressed

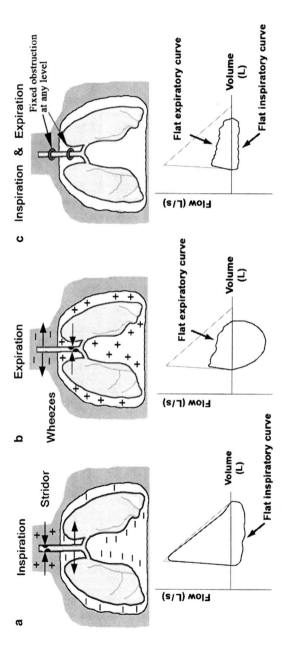

FIGURE 1.20. Upper airway obstruction: (**a**) variable extrathoracic obstruction; (**b**) Variable intrathoracic obstruction; (**c**) Fixed upper airway obstruction.

by the increased intrathoracic pressure that occurs during expiration; Figure 1.20b. A variable lesion, e.g., tracheomalacia, in the upper airways will compress easily when the pressure outside exceeds the pressure inside the airways. Central tumors can also preferentially reduce expiratory flow. In these cases you may hear expiratory wheezes with the stethoscope placed in the midline over the upper chest.

(b) Unlike the obstruction in the lower airways (as in asthma and COPD), the expiratory component of the FV loop in intrathoracic upper airway obstruction is deformed throughout its entire length, starting right from the PEF, which is significantly reduced; Figure 1.20b.

(c) To remember which part of the FV loop is affected by a variable upper airway obstruction, think of the upper airways oriented upside down beside the FV loop with the horizontal (volume) axis at the level of the sternal notch; Figure 1.21. Flattening of the lower part of the loop will then indicate a variable extrathoracic lesion and vice versa; Figure 1.21. This way of remembering the different types of obstruction may sound odd, but with time you will find that it is useful[‖].

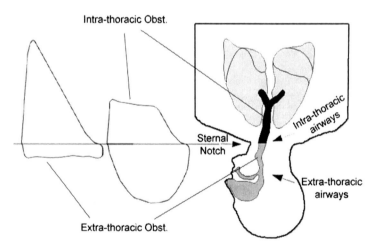

FIGURE 1.21. A way to remember which part of the curve is deformed in either forms of variable upper airway obstruction.

[‖] Another way is to think of the *intra*thoracic obstruction taking place during the *ex*-piration, while the *extra*thoracic during the *in*-spiration. So, intra- will take ex-, while extra- will take in-.

3. *Fixed upper airway obstruction* (above or below the sternal notch)
  (a) This type of obstruction does not change with inspiration or expiration (not dynamic), and hence, it will not matter whether it is located in the intra- or extrathoracic compartment of the upper airways.
  (b) As a result, both the inspiratory and the expiratory components of the FV loop are flattened; Figure 1.20c
  (c) See Table 1.8 for causes of upper airway obstruction.

Note: In the absence of FV loop, you can still identify the different types of upper airway obstruction numerically using PEF, PEF/FEV_1 ratio, FIF_{50}, and FIF_{50}/FEF_{50} ratio; see Table 1.9.**

TABLE 1.8. Causes of upper airway obstruction[8]

Variable extrathoracic lesions (lesions above the sternal notch)
  Dynamic tumors of hypopharynx or upper trachea
  Vocal cord paralysis
  Dynamic subglottic stenosis
  External compression of upper trachea (e.g., by goiter)

Variable intrathoracic lesions (lesions below the sternal notch)
  Dynamic tumors of the lower trachea
  Tracheomalacia
  Dynamic tracheal strictures
  Chronic inflammatory disorders of the upper airways (e.g., Wegener granulomatosis, relapsing polychondritis)
  External compression of lower trachea (e.g., by retrosternal goiter)

Fixed lesions (lesions at any level in the major airways)
  Non-dynamic tumors at any level of upper airways
  Fibrotic stricture of upper airways

TABLE 1.9. Differentiating types of upper airway obstruction numerically[10]

	Fixed UAO	Variable extrathoracic	Variable intrathoracic
PEF	↓	↓ or normal	↓
PEF/FEV_1	Not applicable	<8[47,51]	Not applicable
FIF_{50}	↓	↓	↓ or normal
FIF_{50}/FEF_{50}	~1	<1	>1

_____

**MIF_{50} & MEF_{50} are sometimes used to describe FIF_{50} & FEF_{50}, respectively & they stand for the maximal inspiratory flow at 50% of FIVC and the maximal expiratory flow at 50% of FVC, respectively.

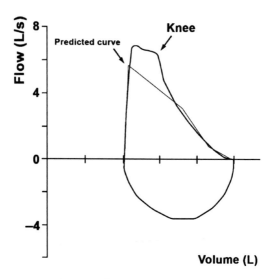

FIGURE 1.22. Normal variant, *knee*. Note that the PEF is normal.

A normal variant that mimics a variable intrathoracic upper airway obstruction; Figure 1.22.
- The key to differentiating this normal variant from a variable intrathoracic upper airway obstruction is the preserved PEF. Although the peak of the FV curve in this condition is flattened suggesting upper airway obstruction, the PEF is actually preserved compared to the predicted curve. In variable intrathoracic upper airway obstruction, PEF is reduced.
- Acceptability criteria may be questioned here (suggesting a poor start); however, when this curve is highly reproducible, it is recognized as a normal variant. This variant is very common and is sometimes referred to as the *knee* variant.[8,22]

References

1. Miller MR, Hankinson J, Brusasco V, et al.. Standardisation of spirometry. Eur Respir J 2005;26:319–338.
2. American Thoracic Society. Standardization of spirometry, 1994 update. Am J Respir Crit Care Med 1995;152:1107–1136.
3. Paoletti P, Pistelli G, Fazzi P, et al.. Reference values for vital capacity and flow–volume curves from a general population study. Bull Eur Physiopathol Respir 1986;22:451–459.
4. Brusasco V, Pellegrino R, Rodarte JR. Vital capacities during acute and chronic bronchoconstriction: dependence on flow and volume histories. Eur Respir J 1997;10:1316–1320.

5. Hansen LM, Pedersen OF, Lyager S, Naerra N. [Differences in vital capacity due to the methods employed]. Ugerkr Laeger 1983;145:2752–2756.

6. Swanney MP, Jensen RL, Crichton DA, Beckert LE, Cardno LA, Crapo RO. FEV(6) is an acceptable surrogate for FVC in the spirometric diagnosis of airway obstruction and restriction. Am J Respir Crit Care Med 2000;162:917–919.

7. Hardie JA, Buist AS, Vollmer WM, Ellingsen I, Bakke PS, Morkve O. Risk of over-diagnosis of COPD in asymptomatic elderly never-smokers. Eur Respir J 2002;20:1117–1122.

8. Hyatt RE, Scanlon PD, Nakamura M. Interpretation of Pulmonary Function Tests: A Practical Guide, 2nd edition. Lippincott Williams & Wilkins, Philadelphia, PA, 2003.

9. Hancox B, Whyte K. Pocket Guide to Lung Function Tests, 1st Edition. McGraw-Hill, Sydney, 2001.

10. Pellegrino R, Viegi G, Enright P, et al. Interpretative strategies for lung function tests. Eur Respir J 2005;26:948–968.

11. Flenley DC. Chronic obstructive pulmonary disease. Dis Mon 1988;34:537–599.

12. Gardner RM, Clausen JL, Crapo RO, et al. Quality assurance in pulmonary function laboratories. Am Rev Respir Dis 1986;134:626–627.

13. Association for the Advancement of Medical Instrumentation, Standard for spirometers (draft), October 1980. AAMI Suite 602, 1901 N. Ft. Myer Drive, Arlington, VA 22209–1699.

14. Miller MR, et al. General considerations for lung function testing. Eur Respir J 2005;26:153–161

15. Renzetti AD Jr. Standardization of spirometry. Am Rev Respir Dis 1979;119:831–838.

16. Morris AH, Kanner RE, Crapo RO, Gardner RM. Clinical pulmonary function testing: a manual of uniform laboratory procedures, 2nd Edition. Intermountain Thoracic Society, Salt Lake City, UT, 1984.

17. Smith AA, Gaensler EA. Timing of forced expiratory volume in one second. Am Rev Respir Dis 1975;112:882–885.

18. Hankinson JL, Gardner RM. Standard waveforms for spirometer testing. Am Rev Respir Dis 1982;126:362–364.

19. Horvath EP Jr, ed. Manual of spirometry in occupational medicine. Division of Training and Manpower Development, National Institutes for Occupational Safety and Health, Cincinnati, OH, 1981.

20. Stoller JK, Basheda S, Laskowski D, Goormastic M, McCarthy K. Trial of standard versus modified expiration to achieve end-of-test spirometry criteria. Am Rev Respir Dis 1993;148:275–280.

21. Townsend MC. The effects of leaks in spirometers on measurement of pulmonary function. J Occup Med 1984;26:835–841.

22. Salzman SH. Pulmonary Function Testing. ACCP Pulmonary Board Review Course, Northbrook, IL, 2005:297–320.

23. Stocks J, Quanjer PH. Reference values for residual volume, functional residual capacity and total lung capacity. ATS Workshop on Lung Volume Measurements. Official Statement of The European Respiratory Society. Eur Respir J 1995;8:492–506.

24. Quanjer PH, Tammeling GJ, Cotes JE, Pedersen OF, Peslin R, Yernault JC. Lung volumes and forced ventilatory flows. Report Working Party Standardization of Lung Function Tests, European Community for Steel and Coal. Official Statement of the European Respiratory Society. Eur Respir J 1993;6 Suppl 16:S5–S40.

25. Cotes JE, Chinn DJ, Quanjer PH, Roca J, Yernault JC. Standardization of the measurement of transfer factor (diffusing capacity). Report Working Party Standardization of Lung Function Tests, European Community for Steel and Coal. Official Statement of the European Respiratory Society. Eur Respir J 1993;6 Suppl 16:S41–S52.

26. Solberg HE, Grasbeck R. Reference values. Adv Clin Chem 1989; 27:1–79.

27. American Thoracic Society. Lung function testing: selection of reference values and interpretative strategies. Am Rev Respir Dis 1991;144:1202–1218.

28. Parker JM, Dillard TA, Phillips YY. Arm span-height relationships in patients referred for spirometry. Am J Respir Crit Care Med 1996;154:533–536.

29. Korotzer B, Ong S, Hansen JE. Ethnic differences in pulmonary function in healthy nonsmoking Asian-Americans and European-Americans. Am J Respir Crit Care Med 2000;161:1101–1108.

30. Sharp DS, Enright PL, Chiu D, Burchfiel CM, Rodriguez BL, Curb JD. Reference values for pulmonary function tests of Japanese-American men aged 71–90 years. Am J Respir Crit Care Med 1996;153:805–811.

31. Pauwels RA, Buist AS, Calverley PM, Jenkins CR, Hurd SS, GOLD Scientific Committee. Global strategy for the diagnosis, management, and prevention of chronic obstructive pulmonary disease. NHLBI/WHO Global Initiative for Chronic Obstructive Lung Disease (GOLD) Workshop summary. Am J Respir Crit Care Med 2001;163:1256–1276.

32. American Thoracic Society. Evaluation of impairment/disability secondary to respiratory disorders. Am Rev Respir Dis 1986;133:1205–1209.

33. American Medical Association. Guides to the Evaluation of Permanent Impairment, 4th Edition. American Medical Association, Chicago, IL, 1995.

34. Aaron SD, Dales RE, Cardinal P. How accurate is spirometry at predicting restrictive impairment. Chest 1999;115:869–873.

35. Glady CA, Aaron SD, Lunau M, Clinch J, Dales RE. A spirometry-based algorithm to direct lung function testing in the pulmonary function laboratory. Chest 2003;123:1939–1946.

36. Guyatt GH, Townsend M, Nogradi S, Pugsley SO, Keller JL, Newhouse MT. Acute response to bronchodilator, an imperfect guide for bronchodilator therapy in chronic airflow limitation. Arch Intern Med 1988;148:1949–1952.

37. Brand PL, Quanjer PhH, Postma DS, et al. Interpretation of bronchodilator response in patients with obstructive airways disease. Thorax 1992;47:429–436.

38. Coates AL, Allen PD, MacNeish CF, Ho SL, Lands LC. Effect of size and disease on expected deposition of drugs administered using jet nebulization in children with cystic fibrosis. Chest 2001;119:1123–1130.

39. Coates AL, Ho SL. Drug administration by jet nebulization. Pediatr Pulmonol 1998;26:412–423.

40. Newman SP, Clark AR, Talaee N, Clark SW. Pressurized aerosol deposition in the human lung with and without an "open" spacer device. Thorax 1989;44:706–710.

41. Tal A, Golan H, Grauer N, Aviram M, Albin D, Quastel MR. Deposition pattern of radiolabeled salbutamol inhaled from a meter-dose inhaler by means of a spacer with mask in young children with airway obstruction. J Pediatr 1996;128:479–484.

42. Newhouse MT. Asthma therapy with aerosols: are nebulizers obsolete? A continuing controversy. J Pediatr 1999;135:5–8.

43. Coates AL, MacNeish CF, Lands LC, Meisner D, Kelemen S, Vadas EB. A comparison of the availability of tobramycin for inhalation from vented versus unvented nebulizers. Chest 1998;113:951–956.

44. Devadason SG, Everard ML, Linto JM, LeSouef PN. Comparison of drug delivery form conventional versus "Venturi" nebulizers. Eur Respir J 1997;10:2479–2483.

45. Leach CL, Davidson PJ, Hasselquist BE, Boudreau RJ. Lung deposition of hydofluoroalkane-134a beclomethasone is greater than that of chlorofluorocarbon fluticasone and chlorofluorocarbon beclomethasone: a cross-over study in healthy volunteers. Chest 2002;122:510–516.

46. Cerveri I, Pellegrino R, Dore R, et al.. Mechanisms for isolated volume response to a bronchodilator in patients with COPD. J Appl Physiol 2000;88:1989–1995.

47. Empey DW. Assessment of upper airways obstruction. BMJ 1972;3:503–505.

48. Bates DV. Respiratory Function in Disease, 3rd Edition. WB Saunders, Philadelphia, 1989.

49. Wilson AF, ed. Pulmonary Function Testing, Indications and Interpretations. Grune & Stratton, Orlando, FL, 1985.

50. Pride NB, Macklem PT. Lung mechanics in disease. In: Macklem PT, Mead J, eds. Handbook of Physiology. The Respiratory System. Mechanics of Breathing. Section 3, Vol. III, Part 2. American Physiological Society, Bethesda, MD, 1986;659–692.

51. Miller MR, Pincock AC, Oates GD, Wilkinson R, Skene-Smith H. Upper airway obstruction due to goitre: detection, prevalence and results of surgical management. Q J Med 1990;74:177–188.

52. Miller RD, Hyatt RE. Obstructing lesions of the larynx and trachea. Mayo Clin Proc 1969;44:145–161.

53. Pedersen OF, Ingram RH Jr. Configuration of maximum expiratory flow–volume curve: model experiments with physiological implications. J Appl Physiol 1985;58:1305–1313.

54. Miller MR, Pedersen OF. Peak flow meter resistance decreases peak expiratory flow in subjects with COPD. J Appl Physiol 2000;89:283–290.

55. Gibson GJ. Central airway obstruction. In: Clinical Tests of Respiratory Function, 2nd Edition. Chapman & Hall, London, 1996;194–202.

56. Lorber DB, Kaltenborn W, Burrows B. Responses to isoproterenol in a general population sample. Am Rev Respir Dis 1978;118:855–861.

Chapter 2
Lung Volumes

Measuring lung volumes helps characterize certain disease states. These volumes are termed the static lung volumes, while spirometry measures the dynamic volumes. This chapter will discuss these lung volumes, how they are measured, and their clinical implications.

DEFINITIONS; SEE FIGURE 2.1

Total lung capacity (TLC)

- Is the volume of air (in liters) that a subject's lungs can contain at the end of a maximal inspiration.[1]

Residual volume (RV)

- Is the volume of air that remains in the lungs at the end of a maximal exhalation.[1] An abnormal increase in RV is called *air trapping*. The techniques used to measure lung volumes are primarily designed to measure the residual volume, as this volume cannot be exhaled to be measured. The rest of the lung volumes can then be measured by simple spirometry, using the SVC rather than the FVC. The TLC can then be calculated by adding RV to VC or *functional residual capacity (FRC)* to *inspiratory capacity (IC)*; Figure 2.1.
- Therefore, spirometry is an essential part of any lung volume study.

A. Altalag et al., *Pulmonary Function Tests in Clinical Practice*,
DOI: 10.1007/978-1-84882-231-3_2, © Springer-Verlag London Limited 2009

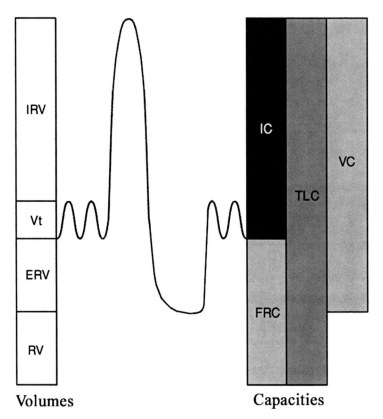

FIGURE 2.1. A volume spirogram showing the different lung volumes (*on the left*) and capacities (*on the right*).

Functional residual capacity

- Is the volume of air that remains in the lungs at the end of a tidal exhalation, i.e., when the respiratory muscles are at rest.[1] This means that at FRC, the resting negative intrathoracic pressure produced by the chest wall (rib cage and diaphragm) wanting to expand is balanced by the elastic recoil force of the lungs, which naturally want to contract. Therefore, when the elastic recoil of the lungs decreases as in emphysema, the FRC increases (hyperinflation), while when the elastic recoil increases as in pulmonary fibrosis, the FRC decreases.
- The FRC is the sum of the *expiratory reserve volume (ERV)* and the RV and is ~50% of TLC.

- FRC measured using body plethysmography (discussed later) is sometimes referred to as the *thoracic gas volume (TGV or V_{TG}) at FRC or V_{FRC}*.[1] Indeed, FRC is the volume measured by all the volume measuring techniques and RV is then determined by subtracting ERV.
- FRC has important functions:
  - Aids the mixed venous blood oxygenation during expiration and before the next inspiration.
  - Decreases the energy required to reinflate the lungs during inspiration. If, for example, each time the patient exhales, the lungs want to go to the fully collapsed position, a tremendous force will be needed to reinflate them. Such effort would soon result in exhaustion and respiratory failure.[2]

Expiratory reserve volume (ERV)

- Is the maximum volume of air that can be exhaled at the end of a tidal exhalation and can be measured by simple spirometry.[1]

Inspiratory reserve volume (IRV)

- Is similarly defined as the maximum volume of air that can be inhaled following a tidal inhalation.[1]

Inspiratory capacity (IC)

- Is the maximum volume of air that can be inhaled after a normal exhalation.[1] Accordingly, IC equals the IRV + tidal volume (V_T).

Tidal volume (V_T)

- Is the volume of air that we normally inhale or exhale while at rest, and equals roughly 0.5 L in an average adult and increases with exercise.

SVC or VC

- Was discussed in Chapter 1. See Figure 2.6.

The Terms "Volume" and "Capacity"; Figure 2.1[3]

- The term "volume" refers to the lung volumes that cannot be broken down into smaller components (RV, ERV, VT, and IRV).

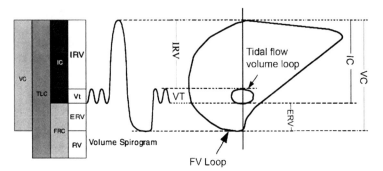

FIGURE 2.2. To aid in understanding lung volumes as they relate to the FV curve, the FV curve may be rotated 90° clockwise and placed beside the volume spirogram.

- The term "capacity" refers to the lung volumes that can be broken down into other smaller components (IC, FVC, TLC, and VC).
  - IC = IRV + VT
  - FVC = ERV + RV
  - VC = IC + ERV
  - TLC = VC + RV

Correlation with the FV Curve

- FV curve can be used as a volume spirogram (seen in Figure 2.1), in addition to its other uses; Figure 2.2. The only three lung volumes that spirometry cannot measure are RV, FRC, and TLC.

METHODS FOR MEASURING THE STATIC LUNG VOLUMES

- There are different ways of measuring the lung volumes, among which the most accurate and widely used is the body box or body plethysmography. The other, less widely used, methods are the nitrogen washout method, the inert gas dilution technique, and the radiographic method.
- This section will discuss the principles, the advantages, and the disadvantages of each method.

Body Plethysmography (Body Box)

- Is an ingenious way of measuring the lung volumes. The primary goal is to measure the FRC by the body box, in addition to allowing measures of the ERV and the SVC. The RV and TLC can then be calculated from these three variables (RV = FRC – ERV; TLC = RV + SVC); see Figure 2.1.

- The principle of body plethysmography depends on *Boyle's law*, which states that the product of pressure and volume of a gas

TABLE 2.1. Principle of body plethesmography[1,4,5,7,8]

The principle of body plethysmography depends on Boyle's law, which states that the product of pressure and volume ($P \times V$) of a gas is constant under constant temperature conditions (which is the case in the lungs):

Therefore: $P_1 \times V_1 = P_2 \times V_2$

The patient is put in the plethysmograph (an airtight box with a known volume), with a clip placed on the nose, and the mouth tightly applied around a mouthpiece; see Figure 2.3. The patient is then instructed to breathe at the resting tidal volume (V_T). The first part of the earlier equation (Boyle's law) can then be applied at the patient's FRC (the end of a normal exhalation), where:

- P_1 is the pressure of air in the lungs at FRC (the beginning of the test), which equals the barometric pressure (760 cmH$_2$O, at sea level).
- V_1 is the FRC (V_{FRC}) that is the volume of air in the lungs at the beginning of the test.

At FRC, a valve (shutter) will close and the patient will perform a panting maneuver through an occluded airway where the change in pressure will be measured (ΔP).

The air in the lungs will get compressed and decompressed as a result of the change in pressure, resulting in a change in lung volume, i.e., a change in FRC (ΔV). We can now apply the new pressure and volume on the second part of the same equation, earlier, where:

- P_2 (the pressure of air in the lungs when the air gets decompressed as a result of the negative pressure produced by the inspiratory muscles during the panting maneuver, after the valve closure) will equal the initial pressure (P_1) minus the change in pressure (ΔP), i.e., $P_2 = (P_1 - \Delta P)$.
- Similarly, V_2 (the volume of air in the lungs after it gets decompressed) will equal the sum of the initial volume of the lung (V_1 or V_{FRC}) plus the change in volume (ΔV).
  So, $V_2 = (V_1 + \Delta V)$
- By substituting these values in the original equation ($P_1 \times V_1 = P_2 \times V_2$), we will get:

(continued)

TABLE 2.1. (continued)

- $P_1 \times V_1 = (P_1 - \Delta P) \times (V_1 + \Delta V)$; multiplying $(P_1 - \Delta P)$ by $(V_1 + \Delta V)$:
- $P_1 \times V_1 = (P_1 \times V_1) + (P_1 \times \Delta V) - (\Delta P \times V_1) - (\Delta P \times \Delta V)$; subtracting $(P_1 \times V_1)$ from both sides:
- $0 = (P_1 \times \Delta V) - (\Delta P \times V_1) - (\Delta P \times \Delta V)$; adding $(\Delta P \times V_1)$ to both sides:
- $(\Delta P \times V_1) = (P_1 \times \Delta V) - (\Delta P \times \Delta V)$; dividing by ΔP
- $(\Delta P \times V_1)/\Delta P = [(P_1 \times \Delta V) - (\Delta P \times \Delta V)]/\Delta P$
  or $V_1 = [\Delta V \times (P_1 - \Delta P)]/\Delta P$
- As ΔP is too small compared with P_1 (20 cmH$_2$O compared with a barometric pressure of 760 cm H$_2$O), then we can accept: $P_1 - \Delta P = P_1$. Then, the final equation can be simplified as follows:
  $V_1 = (\Delta V \times P_1)/\Delta P$ or $V_{FRC} = (\Delta V \times P_1)/\Delta P$; as P_1 is the barometric pressure; each of ΔP and ΔV are measured by the plethysmograph.
- After determining the FRC, the RV and TLC can be calculated, as discussed earlier. You do not need to worry about all of this, as a computer does all the measurements and calculations, but it is still good to know how it does all that.
- In plethysmography, the FRC is sometimes referred to as the thoracic gas volume (TGV or V_{TG}).

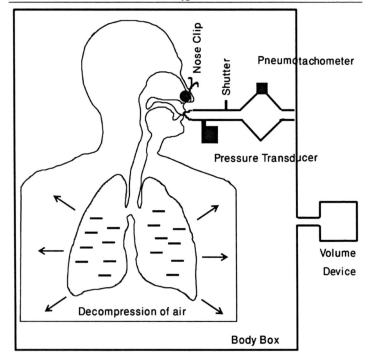

FIGURE 2.3. Principle of body plethesmography (the body box)

is constant at a constant temperature.[4, 5] For the details of how this law is applied in the body box to get the FRC, see Table 2.1 (Figure 2.3).

• The plethysmograph is the most popular way of measuring the lung volumes, as it is the fastest and probably the most accurate, but it is the most expensive too. A comparison between the methods for measuring the lung volumes is shown in Table 2.4.[5,6]

Nitrogen Washout Method[1,9]

• Is another way of determining FRC. This technique is less accurate and more time consuming (at least 7 min[10]). Its principle is related to the concentration of nitrogen in the lungs (which is the concentration of the atmospheric nitrogen, 80%), which then can be washed out to determine the volume. See Table 2.2 (Figure 2.4) for details.

Inert Gas Dilution Technique[1,11,12]

• An inert gas is a gas that is not absorbable in the air spaces. As in N_2 washout method, the inert gas technique is less accurate

TABLE 2.2. Nitrogen washout method[1,9]

At FRC (the end of a normal exhalation), the patient will breathe into a closed system. He/she will inhale 100% O_2 and exhale into a separate container with a known volume. The patient will continue this process, until almost all the nitrogen in the lungs is exhaled into that container. The nitrogen concentration in the container is then determined.

The equation of the concentration (C) and volume (V) can then be applied: $C_1 \times V_1 = C_2 \times V_2$, where:

  ○ C_1 is the N_2 concentration in the lungs at FRC (80%)
  ○ V_1 is the FRC (unknown)
  ○ C_2 is the N_2 concentration in the container (known)
  ○ V_2 is the volume of air in the collecting container (known)

The FRC can then be determined. Keep in mind that two correction factors are made for accurate results. One is to account for the N_2 that remains in the lungs at the end of the test and the second is to account for the N_2 that is continuously released from the circulation into the lungs during the test.

In obstructive disorders, more time (20 min) than usual is needed to washout N_2 from the poorly ventilated areas, resulting in underestimation of the lung volumes. The test is normally terminated after 7 min,[10] while body plethysmography is usually carried out over less than a minute. A significant increase in TLC measured by plethysmography compared with that measured by N_2 washout method suggests air trapping commonly seen in obstructive disorders (COPD).

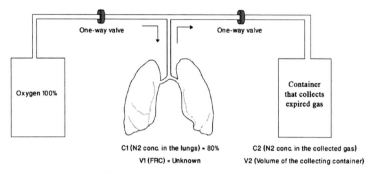

C1 (N2 conc. in the lungs) = 80%   C2 (N2 conc. in the collected gas)
V1 (FRC) = Unknown   V2 (Volume of the collecting container)

FIGURE 2.4. Principle of Nitrogen washout method.

TABLE 2.3. Inert gas dilution technique[1,11,12]

At FRC (the end of a normal exhalation), the patient will breathe into
a closed system with a known volume (V_1) and concentration (C_1) of
an inert gas [helium (He)]. The patient will continue breathing the
helium until concentration equilibrium is reached and measured by
a helium analyzer (C_2). V_2 will be the sum of the original volume of
helium (V_1) and the initial lung volume (FRC).

The equation of the concentration (C) and volume (V) can be applied to
get the FRC as follows:

- $C_1 \times V_1 = C_2 \times V_2$, where $V_2 = (V_1 + \text{FRC})$, therefore:
  $C_1 \times V_1 = C_2 \times (V_1 + \text{FRC})$

  $$\text{FRC} = [(C_1 \times V_1)/C_2] - (V_1)$$
  $$= V_1 \times [(C_1/C_2) - 1] = V_1 \times [(C_1/C_2) - (C_2/C_2)]$$
  $$= V_1 \times (C_1 - C_2)/C_2$$

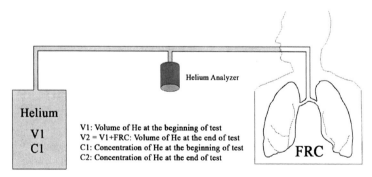

Helium Analyzer

Helium

V1
C1

V1: Volume of He at the beginning of test
V2 = V1+FRC: Volume of He at the end of test
C1: Concentration of He at the beginning of test
C2: Concentration of He at the end of test

FRC

FIGURE 2.5. Principle of Inert Gas (Helium) Dilution Technique.

(underestimates lung volumes in airway obstruction) and is more time consuming. See Table 2.3 (Figure 2.5) for details.

Radiographic Method (Planimetry or Geometry)

- The TLC and RV are estimated by doing posteroanterior (PA) and lateral chest radiographs during full inspiration (TLC) and full expiration (RV). It is an invasive method that is not used routinely, due to the unnecessary exposure to radiation. This method may yield a lower TLC by >10% compared with plethysmography.[14-16] CT scan and MRI are more accurate than plane radiography in determining TLC but they are more costly.[17-19]
- In a normal subject, all the aforementioned methods should give similar values for the lung volumes, if done properly.[1] It is only in disease state, when the values will vary between the different methods; Table 2.4.

TECHNIQUE FOR BODY PLETHYSMOGRAPHY

- The plethysmograph should be calibrated daily to ensure accuracy.[1,20-22] The temperature and barometric pressure should be entered every morning.
- The patient sits comfortably inside the body box, with the door closed, a nose clip applied, and the mouth tightly applied to a mouthpiece.

TABLE 2.4. Comparison between the common methods for measuring lung volumes[5,6]

Plethysmography	N_2 washout method/Inert gas dilution technique
Fast	Time consuming
Readily repeatable for reproducibility	Difficult to repeat.[1,13] The test is too long[1]; more time is required for the lungs to equilibrate and to clear inert gas in the dilution technique.
More accurate	Less accurate
Slightly overestimates FRC in obstructive disorders[5]	Underestimates FRC in obstructive disorders
Difficult to test patients on wheel chairs or stretchers or patients attached to i.v. pumps	Possible to test patients on wheel chairs or stretchers
Expensive, large size, and complex	Cheap and small

- The patient should breathe normally at the V_T until three or four stable tidal breaths are achieved; Figure 2.6. Then (step1) at the end of the last tidal exhalation (FRC), the patient is instructed to pant fast and shallowly[23] against a closed valve (shutter), where the plethysmograph measures the FRC, as explained earlier.
- Step 2: the patient is then instructed to take a full inspiration (IC), then (step 3) deep, slow expiration (SVC or VC) for at least 6 s, which is spirometry. The subsets of lung volumes can then be calculated, as shown in Figure 2.6.*
- The test is then repeated for reproducibility as ATS criteria should also be met in the measurements. The difference between the two measurements of FRC and TLC should be within 10% and RV within 20%.[1]
- Physical and biological calibrations are also needed.
  - The physical calibration is done every morning and includes calibrating the mouth pressure transducer and the volume signal of the plethysmograph. The volume calibration is

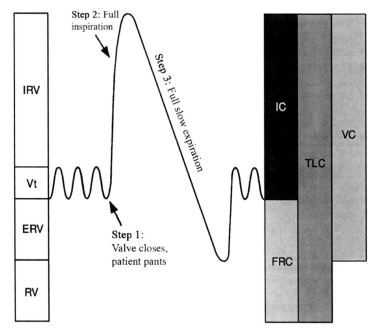

FIGURE 2.6. Technique for plethysmography. Notice that SVC is used instead of FVC.

---

*In some labs, the patient is instructed to exhale fully after the panting maneuver to measure ERV then to inhale fully to measure VC.

carried out using a container with a known volume (a 3-L lung model) where the container's gas volume measurements should be within 50 ml or 3% of each other, whichever is larger.[1,5]

- Biological calibration should be done once a month on two reference subjects.[1] Measurements should not be significantly different from the previously acquired measurements in the same subjects (<10% for TLC and FRC and <20% for RV).[1]

CORRELATING THE FLOW–VOLUME CURVE WITH LUNG VOLUMES

- When the FV curve is done while the patient is inside the body box, at the same time as the lung volume study, the TLC and RV can be accurately plotted on the curve too. As discussed in Chapter 1, TLC is represented by the leftmost point of the curve and RV by the rightmost point of the curve. Comparing these points with their equivalents in the predicted curve will indicate whether these lung volumes are decreased, normal, or increased.
- In restrictive disorders, the TLC and RV are low, which means that the curve will shift to the right compared with the predicted (remember, *r*ight = *r*estrictive). The opposite is true in obstructive disorders; see Figure 2.7.

REFERENCE VALUES[1,24–29]

- As in spirometry, reference values are derived from Caucasian studies, and corrections should be made in non-Caucasians. These reference values are related to body size, with the height being the most important factor. Values above the fifth percentile are considered normal; see Appendix 2.

COMPONENTS OF A LUNG VOLUME STUDY

- The simple rule for lung volumes is that they increase in obstructive disorders and decrease in restrictive disorders. TLC and RV are the most important for interpreting PTFs. The RV/TLC ratio is similarly useful in interpreting lung volume studies. Table 2.5 discusses the causes for abnormal lung volumes. IC and IRV are not discussed as they have little diagnostic role.

CLINICAL SIGNIFICANCE OF FRC

- A high FRC (as in emphysema) means that when the patient is not breathing in, the lungs contain more air than normal.

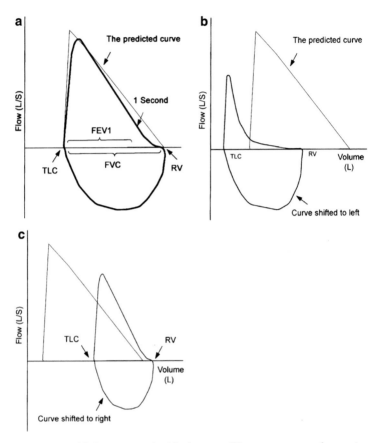

FIGURE 2.7. (a) Represents the ideal curve; (b) represents an obstructive disorder with increased TLC and RV and shift of FV curve to the left; (c) represents a restrictive disorder with decreased TLC and RV and shift of FV curve to the right.

Breathing at that high lung volume helps prevent collapse of the airways and air trapping in emphysematous lungs, but at the same time, increases the effort of breathing. This can be very uncomfortable and can lead to dyspnea. Try that by taking a deep breath and try to talk and breathe at that lung volume and see for yourself. The increased effort noticed when breathing at high lung volumes is caused by two consequences of a high lung volume. Firstly, the breathing muscles are shortened and become at a mechanical disadvantage. As a result, more muscular activity is required to produce the pressure gradient that

TABLE 2.5. Causes of abnormal lung volumes

TLC
Increased in:

- COPD, mainly emphysema
- Acromegaly patients may have a high TLC,[2] which can be differentiated from emphysema by RV/TLC ratio (normal in acromegaly and high in emphysema[31])
- TLC may be high in normal subjects with big lungs, e.g., swimmers
- TLC is usually normal in bronchial asthma, as lung elastic recoil is normal[32]

Decreased in restrictive disorders[30] (see Table 1.7 for classification)

RV
Increased (air trapping) in obstructive disorders:

- COPD
- Bronchial asthma, although the TLC is normal, but the RV is high because of air trapping

Decreased in parenchymal restriction

RV/TLC ratio
Normal in parenchymal restriction[2]
Increased

- Mainly in obstructive disorders[30,31]
- Can be increased in chest wall restriction (because of normal RV and low TLC)

ERV
Decreased in

- Restrictive disorders, similar to TLC
- Obstructive disorders (because of the increased RV due to air trapping that occurs in these conditions)
- An isolated reduction in ERV is characteristic for obesity

FRC
Increased (hyperinflation) in

- Obstructive disorders, mainly emphysema due to loss of lung elastic recoil
- FRC increases slightly with aging

Decreased in

- Restrictive disorders, mainly lung fibrosis
- Obesity
- Supine position (abdominal organs push the diaphragm against the lungs)

leads to airflow and tidal volume. Secondly, the lungs are less compliant as lung volume increases above FRC (more elastic recoil) and so more force is required to produce airflow.

- When patients with emphysema exercise, their respiratory rate increases and the expiratory time decreases. The reduced expiratory time impairs lung emptying and leads to air trapping. The air trapping results in a progressive increase in the FRC with each respiratory cycle. This process continues until the FRC approaches the TLC, at which point, the patient cannot continue exercising. This phenomenon is called *dynamic hyperinflation* and is characteristic of patients with emphysema and is responsible for much of their exercise limitation; Figure 2.8.
- Breathing at a low FRC, as in pulmonary fibrosis and obesity, can also increase the work of breathing. In restrictive lung disorder, the lung compliance is reduced, which means that more effort is needed to inflate the lungs.

DISEASE PATTERNS

The lung volumes are diagnostically useful in many ways. Table 2.6 summarizes their usefulness, which is discussed in more detail in this section:

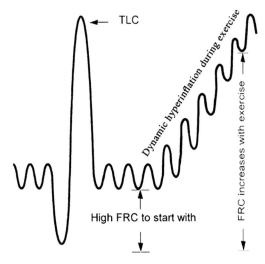

FIGURE 2.8. Dynamic hyperinflation in patients with emphysema during exercise. Note that V_T increases with exercise. Note also that the expiratory phase decreases progressively with continued exercise indicating progressive air trapping.

TABLE 2.6. Additional information acquired by lung volume study compared with spirometry

Differentiates the subtypes of obstructive disorders
Confirms the diagnosis of a restrictive disorder and separates its subtypes
Separates restrictive from obstructive disorders
Helps in detecting combined, obstructive, and restrictive disorders

- *Differentiate subtypes of obstructive disorders*
  - Generally, obstructive disorders (emphysema and asthma) result in increased RV (air trapping) due to airway narrowing while TLC is increased only in emphysema due to loss of elastic recoil. Bronchial asthma, however, has normal elastic recoil and, therefore, normal TLC.[30] As a result, the RV/TLC ratio is increased in both emphysema and bronchial asthma.[31]
  - The RV/TLC ratio can be used also to differentiate an obstructive from a nonobstructive increase in TLC, such as acromegaly (the RV/TLC ratio is normal).[2]
  - If lung volumes are measured pre- and postbronchodilator use, much can be learned from looking at the behavior of TLC and RV before and after the use of bronchodilators. TLC and RV may be shown to decrease following bronchodilators, even in the absence of a significant response in FEV_1 and FVC. Furthermore, IC may increase as FRC may decrease more than TLC in response to bronchodilators. In this case, an increase in IC gives patients with emphysema more room or time to breathe before they develop dynamic hyperinflation to the point of stopping exercise. These volume changes indicate that the bronchodilators are clinically useful to such patients even though there is no change in FEV_1; Figure 2.9.[20,30,33]

- *Confirm the diagnosis of a restrictive disorder* and *differentiate its subtypes*
  - A decreased TLC is essential to make the diagnosis of a restrictive disorder with confidence.[30] The RV and RV/TLC ratio, however, may be used to differentiate the subtypes of restriction:
    - (a) In a parenchymal restriction (lung fibrosis), where there is increased elastic recoil and loss of air space, the RV and

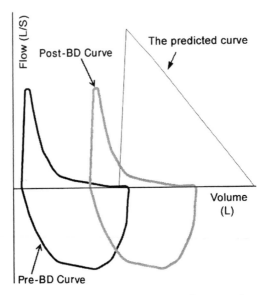

FIGURE 2.9. Post-BD curve is closer to predicted curve indicating significant reduction in TLC and RV compared to that in the pre-BD curve. The
morphology of the curve has not changed indicating no improvement in
FEV_1 or FVC. Despite that BD can be of help to such patients because of
the lung volume change. Note that the change in TLC in this diagram is
exaggerated.

TLC are reduced with a normal RV/TLC ratio (both RV
and TLC decrease proportionately).[2]

(b) In chest wall restriction (NMD, musculoskeletal disease,
paralyzed diaphragms, and obesity), where the lung
parenchyma is normal, the RV is usually normal (or
increased) with an increased RV/TLC ratio (remember
that TLC is low). In NMD, RV may be increased because
the ERV can be very low due to weakness of the expiratory muscles.

(c) The diffusing capacity for carbon monoxide (DL_{CO}) is a
more reliable way of differentiation between parenchymal and chest wall restriction, as will be discussed in the
next chapter. *Maximal voluntary ventilation (MVV)* and
maximal respiratory pressures are measures to help differentiate the different types of chest wall restriction.

  – Obesity and mild bronchial asthma can show a
    spirometric pattern consistent with mild restriction

(decreased FVC and normal FEV_1/FVC ratio), the so-called pseudorestriction. The way to differentiate parenchymal restriction from this pseudorestriction (caused by obesity or mild bronchial asthma) is by the IC/ERV ratio. This ratio is normally 2–3:1. This ratio decreases in parenchymal restriction to <2:1 and increases in pseudorestriction to >6:1. The FV curve (combined with a tidal FV curve) can be used to make that distinction as shown in Figure 2.10.[34]

- Poor patient effort during spirometry may mimic a restrictive disorder, with low FVC and FEV_1 and a normal FEV_1/FVC ratio. In this case a normal TLC can exclude restrictive disorders, as body plethysmography does not require much patient effort. The shape of the FV curve can also easily exclude a poor effort study (PEF is not sharp and is rounded in a poor effort study). In addition, the study is unlikely to be reproducible with a poor effort. The technicians usually indicate in their comments if a poor effort is apparent.

- *Separates obstructive from restrictive disorders*
  - Obstructive and restrictive disorders are sometimes hard to separate based on spirometry alone. Lung volumes may provide additional clues as they are generally increased with obstructive and decreased with restrictive disorders.

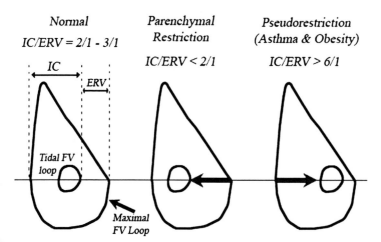

FIGURE 2.10. IC/ERV ratio is used to differentiate parenchymal restriction from pseudorestriction[34].

  – As an example, when the FEV_1 and FVC are at the lower limit
    of the normal range, with a normal FEV_1/FVC ratio, a lung
    volume study may be of value:
    (a) If the TLC and RV are high, then an obstructive disorder
        is the most likely (RV/TLC ratio is usually high).
    (b) If the TLC is normal and RV is mildly increased, then a mild
        bronchial asthma and air trapping could be responsible
        (RV/TLC ratio is high).[2] In this case, the airway obstruc-
        tion is not severe enough to cause significant drop in
        FEV_1 and the ratio. A bronchodilator study may show a
        significant response.
    (c) If the TLC is low, then a restrictive defect is likely to be
        the cause, provided that FVC is below the 5th percentile
        (a normal FVC rules out restriction[36,37]). Before you make
        such a conclusion, have a quick look at the FV curve and
        the rest of the PFT values. If all the values are decreased
        proportionately with a normal FV curve, then consider in
        your report a normal person with relatively small lungs
        (racial variations).
    (d) If the TLC and RV are normal, then the study is most
        likely normal.
- *Detection of combined disorders*
  – Combined disorders are hard to diagnose based on spirom-
    etry alone. Spirometry coupled with a lung volume study is
    very useful:
    (a) An obstructive disorder should be clear in spirometry,
        with low FEV_1/FVC ratio. If this airflow obstruction is
        seen with a reduced TLC, then the reduced TLC suggests
        an additional restrictive disorder.[30,35] The RV could be
        low, normal, or high as airway obstruction may result in
        air trapping and increased RV.[1]
  – Combined defects can be seen in conditions such as sarcoido-
    sis or coexisting COPD and lung fibrosis.
  – Keep in mind that an obstructive disorder (such as emphy-
    sema) with pulmonary resection (lobectomy or pneumonec-
    tomy) can give a similar pattern.
- Chapter 6 discusses the approach to such PFTs in detail.

References

1. Wanger J, Clausen JL, Coates A, et al. Standardisation of the measurement of lung volumes. Eur Respir J 2005;26:511–522.
2. Hyatt RE, Scanlon PD, Nakamura M. Interpretation of Pulmonary
   Function Tests, A Practical Guide, Second Edition. Lippincott Williams
   & Wilkins, Philadelphia, PA, 2003.

3. Salzman SH. Pulmonary Function Testing. ACCP Pulmonary Board Review Course, Northbrook, IL, 2005:297–320.

4. DuBois AB, Botelho SY, Bedell GN, Marshall R, Comroe JH. A rapid plethysmographic method for measuring thoracic gas volume: a comparison with a nitrogen washout method for measuring functional residual capacity in normal subjects. J Clin Invest 1956;35:322–326.

5. Coates AL, Peslin R, Rodenstein D, Stocks J. Measurement of lung volumes by plethysmography. Eur Respir J 1997;10:1415–1427.

6. Stocks J, Quanjer PH. Reference values for residual volume, functional residual capacity and total lung capacity. ATS Workshop on Lung Volume Measurements. Official Statement of the European Respiratory Society. Eur Respir J 1995;8:492–506.

7. NHLBI Workshop. Consensus statement on measurement of lung volumes in humans. www.thoracic.org/adobe/lungvolume.pdf. Date last updated: December 30, 2003. Accessed on July 19, 2005.

8. Madama VC. Pulmonary Function Testing and Cardiopulmonary Stress Testing, First edition. Delmar, Florence, KY, 1993.

9. Newth CJ, Enright P, Johnson RL Jr. Multiple breath nitrogen washout techniques: including measurements with patients on ventilators. Eur Respir J 1997;10:2174–2185.

10. Cournand A, Baldwin ED, Darling RC, Richards DWJ. Studies on intrapulmonary mixture of gases. IV. The significance of the pulmonary emptying rate and a simplified open circuit measurement of residual air. J Clin Invest 1941;20:681–689.

11. Meneely GR, Kaltreider NL. The volume of the lung determined by helium dilution. Description of the method and comparison with other procedures. J Clin Invest 1948;28:129–139.

12. Corbeel LJ. International symposium on body plethysmography. Comparison between measurements of functional residual capacity and thoracic gas volume in chronic obstructive pulmonary disease. Prog Respir Res 1969;4:194–204.

13. Emmanuel G, Briscoe WA, Cournand A. A method for the determination of the volume of air in the lungs: measurement in chronic obstructive pulmonary emphysema. J Clin Invest 1960;20:329–337.

14. Estimation of lung volumes from chest radiographs. In: Clausen JL, ed. Pulmonary Function Testing. Guidelines and Controversies, Equipment, Methods, and Normal Values. Academic, New York, 1982;155–163.

15. Crapo RO, Montague T, Armstrong JD. Inspiratory lung volumes achieved on routine chest films. Invest Radiol 1979;14:137–140.

16. Kilburn KH, Warshaw RH, Thornton JC, Thornton K, Miller A. Predictive equations for total lung capacity and residual volume calculated from radiographs in a random sample of the Michigan population. Thorax 1992;47:518–523.

17. Coxon HO, Hogg JC, Mayo JR, et al. Quantification of idiopathic pulmonary fibrosis using computed tomography and histology. Am J Respir Crit Care Med 1997;155:1649–1656.

18. Johnson RL Jr, Cassidy SS, Grover R, et al. Effect of pneumonectomy on the remaining lung in dogs. J Appl Physiol 1991;70:849–858.

19. Archer DC, Coblenz CL, deKemp RA, Nahnmias C, Norman G. Automated in vivo quantification of emphysema. Radiology 1993;188:835–838.

20. Miller MR, Hankinson J, Brusasco V, et al. Standardisation of spirometry. Eur Respir J 2005;26:319–338.

21. Quanjer PH, Tammeling GJ, Cotes JE, Pedersen OF, Peslin R, Yernault JC. Lung volumes and forced ventilatory flows. Report Working Party, Standardization of Lung Function Tests, European Community for Steel and Coal and European Respiratory Society. Eur Respir J 1993;6 Suppl 16:5–40.

22. American Thoracic Society. Standardization of spirometry. 1994 Update. Am J Respir Crit Care Med 1995;152:1107–1136.

23. Shore SA, Huk O, Mannix S, Martin JG. Effect of panting frequency on the plethysmographic determination of thoracic gas volume in chronic obstructive pulmonary disease. Am Rev Respir Dis 1983;128:54–59.

24. Pellegrino R, Viegi G, Enright P, et al. Interpretative strategies for lung function tests. Eur Respir J 2005;26:948–968.

25. Stocks J, Quanjer PH. Reference values for residual volume, functional residual capacity and total lung capacity. ATS Workshop on Lung Volume Measurements. Official Statement of the European Respiratory Society. Eur Respir J 1995;8:492–506.

26. Quanjer PH, Tammeling GJ, Cotes JE, Pedersen OF, Peslin R, Yernault JC. Lung volumes and forced ventilatory flows. Report Working Party Standardization of Lung Function Tests, European Community for Steel and Coal. Official Statement of the European Respiratory Society. Eur Respir J 1993;6 Suppl 16:S5–S40.

27. Cotes JE, Chinn DJ, Quanjer PH, Roca J, Yernault JC. Standardization of the measurement of transfer factor (diffusing capacity). Report Working Party Standardization of Lung Function Tests, European Community for Steel and Coal. Official Statement of the European Respiratory Society. Eur Respir J 1993;6 Suppl 16:S41–S52.

28. Solberg HE, Grasbeck R. Reference values. Adv Clin Chem 1989;27:1–79.

29. American Thoracic Society. Lung function testing: selection of reference values and interpretative strategies. Am Rev Respir Dis 1991;144:1202–1218.

30. Pellegrino R, Viegi G, Enright P, et al. Interpretative strategies for lung function tests. Eur Respir J 2005;26:948–968.

31. Pride NB, Macklem PT. Lung mechanics in disease. In: Macklem PT, Mead J, eds. Handbook of Physiology. The Respiratory System. Mechanics of Breathing. Section 3, Vol. III, Part 2. American Physiological Society, Bethesda, MD, 1986;659–692.

32. Pride NB. Physiology. In: Clark TJH, Godfrey S, Lee TH, eds. Asthma, Third Edition. Chapman and Hall, London, 1992:14–72.

33. Pellegrino R, Rodarte JR, Brusasco V. Assessing the reversibility of airway obstruction. Chest 1998;114:1607–1612.

34. Salzman S. Pulmonary function testing. Tips on how to interpret the results. J Respir Dis 1999;20:809–822.

35. Dykstra BJ, Scanlon PD, Kester MM, Beck KC, Enright PL. Lung volumes in 4774 patients with obstructive lung disease. Chest 1999; 115:68–74.

36. Aaron SD, Dales RE, Cardinal P. How accurate is spirometry at predicting restrictive impairment. Chest 1999;115:869–873.
37. Glady CA, Aaron SD, Lunau M, Clinch J, Dales RE. A spirometry-based algorithm to direct lung function testing in the pulmonary function laboratory. Chest 2003;123:1939–1946.

Chapter 3
Gas Transfer

DEFINITIONS

Diffusing Capacity for Carbon Monoxide

- Reflects the ability of carbon monoxide (CO) to diffuse into the blood through the alveolar capillary membrane. DL_{CO} is used to estimate gas transfer, which is impaired in many disorders. DL_{CO} stands for *lung diffusing capacity for carbon monoxide* and its traditional unit is ml/min/mmHg.[*,1]
- CO is diffusion-limited as it is highly soluble and strongly binds to Hgb (CO affinity for Hgb is >200 times that for O_2). This feature makes the capillary backpressure for CO very low (almost zero), which allows the gas to diffuse freely to the capillary blood. Therefore, DL_{CO} measurement reflects the diffusing ability of the alveolo-capillary membrane of the lung. A perfusion-limited gas such as acetylene, on the other hand, is so insoluble that if a small fraction of it diffuses to the capillary blood, no more diffusion will take place (no gradient for diffusion) until the capillary blood is replaced by fresh blood (perfusion-limited). This property makes this gas useful in measuring the total pulmonary capillary blood flow (generally reflects the cardiac output) but not diffusion. Oxygen is both diffusion- and

---

[*] In UK and Europe, TL_{CO} is used instead of DL_{CO} and stands for lung transfer factor for carbon monoxide and is expressed in SI units (mmol/min/Kilopascal).[1]

A. Altalag et al., *Pulmonary Function Tests in Clinical Practice*,
DOI: 10.1007/978-1-84882-231-3_3, © Springer-Verlag London Limited 2009

perfusion-limited; therefore, it is not suitable to measure the diffusing capacity.[2]

- DL_{CO} measurement is very reliable and sensitive. As an example, in interstitial lung disorders (ILD), the DL_{CO} level usually decreases before any drop in lung volume. Therefore, DL_{CO} may drop before the disease is obvious clinically or even radiologically. This ability makes it of great value in the diagnosis and follow-up of such conditions.

- DL_{CO} is determined by the amount of blood recruited in the alveolar capillary bed and the alveolo-capillary surface area available for diffusion.

Alveolar Volume (V_A)

- Represents an estimate of the TLC using a single-breath inert gas dilution technique, discussed in the previous chapter. V_A is measured simultaneously with the DL_{CO} measurement using a single-breath technique, which makes it less accurate in estimating the TLC than the standard test.[3,4] (The standard inert gas dilution technique is performed over several minutes that are required for equilibration of the test gas). The result is expressed as "alveolar volume" (V_A) rather than TLC, and V_A should be less than TLC, because in this technique, there is less time for equilibration, and so TLC is underestimated.

- The inert (nonabsorbable) gas used in this test is usually Helium (He), which serves three important roles[†]:
  - Helium is used as an inert gas to calculate the initial alveolar CO concentration prior to diffusion of CO from the alveolar gas.
  - V_A calculated by He dilution corrects DL_{CO} to the actual alveolar volume available for diffusion, a ratio represented as DL_{CO}/V_A.
  - A third indirect use of V_A is to roughly estimate the poorly ventilated volume of the lungs by subtracting V_A from TLC (measured by body plethysmography).

[†]Newer equipment use methane (CH_4) instead of helium as it can be continuously analyzed together with CO using rapidly responding infrared gas analyzers.

TECHNIQUE[1]

- The most popular method of measuring DL_{CO} is the single-breath technique, which is discussed here.[‡] Other methods may be used to measure DL_{CO} but they are less popular (e.g., steady-state, intrabreath, and rebreathing techniques).
- The equipment used to measure DL_{CO} should be calibrated every morning to ensure accuracy.[5,6]
- Technique: After a full exhalation, the patient inhales a mixture of CO, He, O_2, and N_2, each with a known concentration. The patient has to inhale to at least 85% of the previously measured VC, and this will be recorded in the study as inspiratory vital capacity (IVC).[§,7] Then, the patient should hold his/her breath for 10 s to allow for diffusion.[8] This step is critical, as the patient is instructed to keep a neutral pressure on a closed glottis. Blowing out (*Valsalva maneuver*) or sucking in (*Muller maneuver*) during this phase interferes with the results by altering pulmonary blood volume. After the 10-second breath hold, the patient exhales into the machine until a mid-exhalation (representing the alveolar gas) sample is analyzed for the concentration of both, CO & He, Figure 3.1. A mid-exhalation sample is required to avoid sampling the dead space gas.
- The actual duration of breath-hold is recorded in the final report as *breath-hold time* (BHT), in seconds.
- The test is repeated once more (after 4 minutes)[1] for reproducibility & the results should lie within 10% or 3 ml/min/mmHg of each other.[1,9] The maximum number of trials is 5, as following that, the retained CO in the blood from the previous trials will significantly interfere with test results.[¶,1] Don't worry about poisoning the patient with CO, as the amount used for the test is too small, only 0.3% of the gas mixture.[1]
- For details of DL_{CO} calculation using single-breath technique; see Table 3.1.

[‡] The three-equation method is a widely used way of calculating DL_{CO} in the single-breath technique. It is available in some of the newer DL_{CO} measuring devices and probably provides a more accurate measurement.[15]

[§] For most DL_{CO} measuring devices, a VC of at least 1 L is required to produce an accurate measurement of DL_{CO}.

[¶] Five consecutive DL_{CO} measurements may increase CO-Hgb by ~3.5% (i.e., 0.7% per test), which will decrease the measured DL_{CO} by ~3–3.5%.[55]

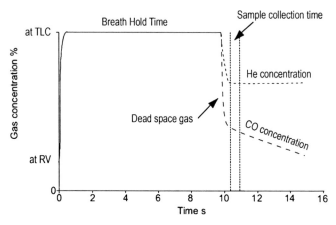

FIGURE 3.1. Schematic of gas concentration during single-breath DL_{CO} measurement. Notice that sample collection takes place after dead-space gas is exhaled (Modified from MacIntyre.[1] With permission.).

TABLE 3.1. Calculating DL_{CO} using single-breath technique[1]

The diffusing capacity for CO (DL_{CO}) equals the rate of CO uptake (Vco) divided by its transfer pressure gradient ($P_ACO - P_cCO$), as P_ACO is the partial pressure of alveolar CO and P_cCO is the mean capillary partial pressure of CO. This relation can be written as follows:

$$DL_{CO} = Vco/(P_ACO - P_cCO)$$

Because P_cCO is negligible as CO almost completely binds to Hgb, the equation can be simplified as follows:

$$DL_{CO} = Vco/P_ACO$$

Vco can be calculated from the difference between the initial and the final CO concentration. Dividing by the logarithmic mean of P_ACO results in the following equation:

$$DL_{CO} = V_A/[T \times (P_B - 47] \times Ln(F_ACO_I/F_ACO_F)$$

as F_ACO_I is the initial alveolar CO concentration (before diffusion), F_ACO_F is the final alveolar CO concentration (after diffusion), T is the breath-hold time (BHT) in minutes, P_B is the barometric pressure, and 47 is the partial pressure of water vapor at body temperature. V_A is the alveolar volume measured by the single-breath helium dilution.

F_ACO_F is measured directly from the mid-exhalation breath sample (alveolar sample after discarding the dead-space washout, 0.7–1.0 L), while F_ACO_I is calculated using the inert gas (He) measurements as follows:

$$F_ACO_I = F_ICO \times (F_AHe/F_IHe)$$

as F_ICO is the inspired CO concentration, F_IHe is the inspired He concentration, and F_AHe is the expired alveolar He concentration, which are all known.

REFERENCE VALUES[10-13]

- Are derived from Caucasian studies. The range (75–120% of the predicted value) is usually accepted as normal for DL_{CO}.** On average, DL_{CO} equals around 25 ml/min/mmHg.

DL_{CO} ADJUSTMENTS

- Adjustment for alveolar volume (V_A)[1,7,14]
  - As discussed earlier, DL_{CO} can be adjusted for V_A (DL_{CO}/V_A ratio). In simple terms, DL_{CO}/V_A represents the diffusing capacity in the available alveolar spaces. In other words, DL_{CO}/V_A determines whether the currently available alveolar spaces are functioning normally.
  - As an example, in patients who had lobectomy or pneumonectomy with an otherwise normal remaining lung tissue, the absolute value for DL_{CO} is expected to be reduced compared with the predicted values. If DL_{CO} is then corrected for V_A (i.e., DL_{CO}/V_A), it will be normal or even high.[1] Therefore, a normal or high DL_{CO}/V_A indicates that the remaining lung tissue is functioning normally. The elevated DL_{CO}/V_A in these patients is due to the increased blood flow in the remaining lung tissue.[1]
  - DL_{CO} is usually reduced in ILD, but, at the same time, V_A is likely to be reduced too in such conditions (due to loss of lung tissue because of fibrosis), which may result in a normal DL_{CO}/V_A. Accordingly, a normal DL_{CO}/V_A cannot exclude ILD. A decreased DL_{CO}/V_A, however, strongly suggests parenchymal lung disease (ILD, emphysema) or pulmonary vascular disease (pulmonary hypertension). A decreased DL_{CO}/V_A is also seen in patients with anemia, as is discussed later. See Chapter 6 for more details for the interpretation of abnormal DL_{CO} measurements.
- Adjustment to Hgb[1,16-20]
  - Anemia results in underestimation of DL_{CO} because of the decreased Hgb available to uptake CO in the pulmonary capillary bed. If the Hgb is not known, anemia should be considered as a possible cause of any isolated or unexplained reduction in DL_{CO}. Similarly, polycythemia will then overestimate DL_{CO}.
  - Correcting DL_{CO} for Hgb is then essential for patients with anemia. The relation between Hgb level and DL_{CO} value

---

**LLN can be applied to appropriate reference equations to determine an abnormal result.

is not a linear relation. For example, if the Hgb is 3 g/dl less than normal, the DL_{CO} drops by ~10%, while if Hgb is 6 g/dl less than normal, the DL_{CO} drops by ~30%.[21] Luckily, there are equations to correct DL_{CO} for Hgb, and in fact, a computer program does all the calculations if the Hgb value is entered. These equations are summarized in Table 3.2.

– A rough way of quickly correcting DL_{CO} for Hgb is by increasing the measured DL_{CO} value by 4% for each 1 g/dl drop from the average (~14.5 for men and ~13.5 for women), and decreasing the measured DL_{CO} by 2% for each g/dl increase in Hgb from the reference (normal) levels.[22]

- Adjustment to carboxy-Hgb (CO-Hgb)
  – Increased CO-Hgb level tends to underestimate the DL_{CO} because of (1) backpressure exerted by the CO-Hgb on the alveolar CO and (2) occupying Hgb binding sites producing an "anemia effect," which results in a reduction in the amount of CO diffusing to the blood.[23–25] Patients who are suspected of smoking prior to the test can have their CO-Hgb levels measured. Once the CO-Hgb level is known the DL_{CO} can be easily estimated by decreasing the predicted DL_{CO} by 1% for each 1% increase in the CO-Hgb level above 2%.[1,26,27] Other more complicated equations may be used.[||]
  – In healthy nonsmokers, CO-Hgb level is ~1–2%, which is acquired from metabolic and environmental sources.[1]
  – Average smokers have a CO-Hgb level of ~4 or 5%, but this can be as high as 10% in heavy smokers.[21] This is why smokers are advised to refrain from smoking for at least 8–10 h and preferably 24 h before the test, but will they comply? Some laboratories do measure the serum CO-Hgb level before DL_{CO} measurement to be certain about the level.

TABLE 3.2. DL_{CO} adjustment to Hgb

Men (adjust to a Hgb value of 14.6 g/dl)[1]

DL_{CO} adj = measured $DL_{CO} \times [(10.22 + Hgb)/(1.7 \times Hgb)]$

Women and children <15 years of age (adjust to a Hgb value of 13.4 g/dl)[1]

DL_{CO} adj = measured $DL_{CO} \times [(9.38 + Hgb)/(1.7 \times Hgb)]$

[||] Alveolar [CO] = (CO-Hgb/O_2Hgb) × [(alveolar [O_2])/210][25,28–30]; DL_{CO} predicted for CO-Hgb = DL_{CO} predicted × (102% – CO-Hgb%).[1]

CAUSES OF ABNORMAL DL$_{CO}$

- Anything that increases the blood flow or volume in the pulmonary capillary bed will result in elevation of DL$_{CO}$. A decreased DL$_{CO}$, however, could be related to either reduced surface area of the lung available for diffusion or disease of the alveolar-capillary membrane. Table 3.3 summarizes the most important causes of abnormal DL$_{CO}$.
- Grading of severity for a reduced DL$_{CO}$ is shown in Table 3.4.

TABLE 3.3. Causes of abnormal DL$_{CO}$

Causes of high DL$_{CO}$
Recruitment of blood in the alveolar capillary bed
    Supine position[1,31–33]
    Hyperdynamic circulation (exercise[31,33,34] and fever)
    Bronchial asthma[35]
    Muller maneuver (inhaling against a closed glottis)[36–38]
    Cardiac causes
        Left to right cardiac shunting[1]
        Early congestive heart failure
Miscellaneous conditions
    Polycythemia[1]
    Alveolar hemorrhage (blood in alveolar space will take up CO)[39]
    Obesity (uncertain mechanism)[40]
    High altitude (due to a lower P_IO_2 at altitude increasing the CO binding to Hgb)[1]
    Following bronchodilators in obstructive disorders (up to 6% increase)[41,42]
    Incorrect reference values

Causes of low DL$_{CO}$
Decreased surface area available for diffusion
    Pulmonary resection (remaining lung tissue will have more blood supply (i.e., $\uparrow$ DL$_{CO}$/V_A) but the overall DL$_{CO}$ will be low)[1]
    Emphysema[43–47] (actual functional alveolo-capillary surface area is reduced)
    VQ mismatch (e.g., significant bronchial obstruction)[1]
Alveolo-capillary membrane disease
    ILD[48,49] (IPF, connective tissue disease, sarcoidosis, hypersensitivity pneumonitis, drugs)
    Pulmonary vascular disease, e.g., pulmonary hypertension or acute pulmonary embolism[1]

(continued)

TABLE 3.3. (continued)

Diffuse alveolar congestion[1,50]
   Late CHF (pulmonary edema fluid impairs gas transfer)
   Diffuse consolidation
   Alveolar proteinosis
Miscellaneous
   Anemia[16–20]
   Elevated CO-Hgb[23–27]
   Pregnancy (unknown mechanism, ~15% drop)[22,50]
   Valsalva maneuver[36,37] (exhaling against closed glottis, opposite to
      Muller maneuver → reduces amount of blood at the capillary bed
      available for diffusion)
   Extrapulmonary reduction in lung inflation (as low effort, NMD, or
      skeletal deformity as in kyphoscoliosis)[1]
   Incorrect reference values
   Others (diurnal variation: lower DL_{CO} by evening,[51,52] during menstrual
      cycle,[53] ingestion of ethanol[54])

TABLE 3.4. Degree of severity of the reduction in diffusing capacity of CO[12]

Degree of severity	DL_{CO} (% pred.)
Mild	60–75%
Moderate	40–60%
Severe	<40%

References

1. MacIntyre N, Crapo RO, Viegi G, et al. Standardisation of the single-breath determination of carbon monoxide uptake in the lung. Eur Respir J 2005;26:720–735.
2. West JB. Respiratory Medicine, the Essentials, Seventh Edition. Lippincott Williams & Wilkins, Philadelphia, PA, 2004.
3. Rodenstein DO, Stanescu DC. Reassessment of lung volume measurement by helium dilution and body plethysmography in COPD. Am Rev Respir Dis 1983;128:54–59.
4. Ferris BG. Epidemiology standardization project (American Thoracic Society). Am Rev Respir Dis 1978;118:1–120.
5. Renzetti AD Jr. Standardization of spirometry. Am Rev Respir Dis 1979;119:831–838.
6. Miller MR, Hankinson J, Brusasco V, et al. Standardisation of spirometry. Eur Respir J 2005;26:319–338.
7. Johnson DC. Importance of adjusting carbon monoxide diffusing capacity (DLCO) and carbon monoxide transfer coefficient (KCO) for alveolar volume. Respir Med 2000;94:28–37.
8. Welle I, Eide GE, Bakke P, Gulsvik A. Applicability of the single-breath carbon monoxide diffusing capacity in a Norwegian community study. Am J Respir Crit Care Med 1998;158:1745–1750.
9. Punjabi NM, Shade D, Patel AM, Wise RA. Measurement variability in single breath diffusing capacity of the lung. Chest 2003;123:1082–1089.

10. Cotes JE, Chinn DJ, Quanjer PH, Roca J, Yernault JC. Standardization of the measurement of transfer factor (diffusing capacity). Report Working Party Standardization of Lung Function Tests, European Community for Steel and Coal. Official Statement of the European Respiratory Society. Eur Respir J 1993;6 Suppl 16:S41–S52.

11. American Thoracic Society. Lung function testing: selection of reference values and interpretative strategies. Am Rev Respir Dis 1991;144:1202–1218.

12. Pellegrino R, Viegi G, Enright P, et al. Interpretative strategies for lung function tests. Eur Respir J 2005;26:948–968.

13. Solberg HE, Grasbeck R. Reference values. Adv Clin Chem 1989;27:1–79.

14. Stam H, Versprille A, Bogaard JM. The components of the carbon monoxide diffusing capacity in man dependent on alveolar volume. Bull Eur Physiopath Respir 1983;19:17–22.

15. Graham BL, Mink JT, Cotton DJ. Effect of breath-hold time on DLCO (SB) in patients with airway obstruction. J Appl Physiol 1985;58:1319–1325.

16. Viegi G, Baldi S, Begliomini E, Ferdeghini EM, Pistelli F. Single breath diffusing capacity for carbon monoxide: effects of adjustment for inspired volume dead space, carbon dioxide, hemoglobin and carboxy-hemoglobin. Respiration 1998;65:56–62.

17. Mohsenifar Z, Brown HV, Schnitzer B, Prause JA, Koerner SK. The effect of abnormal levels of hematocrit on the single breath diffusing capacity. Lung 1982;160:325–330.

18. Clark EH, Woods RL, Hughes JMB. Effect of blood transfusion on the carbon monoxide transfer factor of the lung in man. Clin Sci 1978;54:627–631.

19. Cotes JE, Dabbs JM, Elwood PC, Hall AM, McDonald A, Saunders MJ. Iron-deficiency anaemia: its effect on transfer factor for the lung (diffusing capacity) and ventilation and cardiac frequency during submaximal exercise. Clin Sci 1972;42:325–335.

20. Marrades RM, Diaz O, Roca J, et al. Adjustment of DLCO for hemoglobin concentration. Am J Respir Crit Care Med 1997;155:236–241.

21. Salzman SH. Pulmonary Function Testing. ACCP Pulmonary Board Review Course, Northbrook, IL, 2005:297–320.

22. Hancox B, Whyte K. Pocket Guide to Lung Function Tests, First Edition. McGraw-Hill, Sydney, 2001.

23. Coburn RF, Forster RE, Kane PB. Considerations of the physiological variables that determine the blood carboxyhemoglobin concentration in man. J Clin Invest 1965;44:1899–1910.

24. Viegi G, Paoletti P, Carrozzi L, et al. CO diffusing capacity in a general population sample: relationship with cigarette smoking and air-flow obstruction. Respiration 1993;60:155–161.

25. Mohsenifar Z, Tashkin DP. Effect of carboxyhemoglobin on the single breath diffusing capacity: derivation of an empirical correction factor. Respiration 1979;37:185–191.

26. Comroe JH Jr. Pulmonary diffusing capacity for carbon monoxide (DLCO). Am Rev Respir Dis 1975;111:225–240.

27. Roughton FJW, Forster RE. Relative importance of diffusion and chemical reaction rates in determining rate of exchange of gases in the human lung, with special reference to true diffusing capacity of pulmonary membrane and volume of blood in the lung capillaries. J Appl Physiol 1957;11:290–302.

28. Gaensler EA, Cadigan JB, Ellicott MF, Jones RH, Marks A. A new method for rapid precise determination of carbon monoxide in blood. J Lab Clin Med 1957;49:945–957.

29. Henderson M, Apthorp CH. Rapid method for estimation of carbon monoxide in blood. Br Med J 1960;2:1853–1854.

30. Jones RH, Ellicott MF, Cadigan JB, Gaensler EA. The relationship between alveolar and blood carbon monoxide concentrations during breath-holding. J Lab Clin Med 1958;51:553–564.

31. Huang YC, Helms MI, MacIntyre NR. Normal values for single exhalation diffusing capacity and pulmonary capillary blood flow in sitting, supine positions and during mild exercise. Chest 1994;105:501–508.

32. Stam H, Kreuzer FJA, Versprille A. Effect of lung volume and positional changes on pulmonary diffusing capacity and its components. J Appl Physiol 1991;71:1477–1488.

33. Stokes DL, MacIntyre NR, Nadel JA. Non-linear increases in diffusing capacity during exercise by seated and supine subjects. J Appl Physiol 1981;51:858–863.

34. Johnson RL, Spicer WS, Bishop JM, Forster RE. Pulmonary capillary blood volume, flow and diffusing capacity during exercise. J Appl Physiol 1960;15:893–902.

35. Collard P, Njinou B, Nejadnik B, Keyeux A, Frans A. DLCO in stable asthma. Chest 1994;105:1426–1429.

36. Smith TC, Rankin J. Pulmonary diffusing capacity and the capillary bed during Valsalva and Muller maneuvers. J Appl Physiol 1969;27:826–833.

37. Cotes JE, Snidal DP, Shepard RH. Effect of negative intraalveolar pressure on pulmonary diffusing capacity. J Appl Physiol 1960;15:372–376.

38. Cotton DJ, Mink JT, Graham BL. Effect of high negative inspiratory pressure on single breath CO diffusing capacity. Respir Physiol 1983;54:19–29.

39. Greening AP, Hughes JMB. Serial estimations of DLCO in intrapulmonary hemorrhage. Clin Sci 1981;60:507–512.

40. Collard P, Wilputte JY, Aubert G, Rodenstein DO, Frans A. The DLCO in obstructive sleep apnea and obesity. Chest 1996;110:1189–1193.

41. Iversen ET, Sorensen T, Heckscher T, Jensen JI. Effect of terbutaline on exercise capacity and pulmonary function in patients with chronic obstructive pulmonary disease. Lung 1999;177:263–271.

42. Chinn DJ, Askew J, Rowley L, Cotes JE. Measurement technique influences the response of transfer factor (TLCO) to salbutamol in patients with airflow obstruction. Eur Respir J 1988;1:15–21.

43. Cotton DJ, Prabhu MB, Mink JT, Graham BL. Effects of ventilation inhomogeneity on DLCO SB-3EQ in normal subjects. J Appl Physiol 1992;73:2623–2630.

44. Cotton DJ, Prabhu MB, Mink JT, Graham BL. Effect of ventilation inhomogeneity on "intrabreath" measurements of diffusing capacity in normal subjects. J Appl Physiol 1993;75:927–932.

45. Gelb AF, Gold WM, Wright RR, Bruch HR, Nadel JA. Physiologic diagnosis of subclinical emphysema. Am Rev Respir Dis 1973;107:50–63.

46. Morrison NJ, Abboud RT, Ramadan F, et al. Comparison of single breath carbon monoxide diffusing capacity and pressure–volume curves in detecting emphysema. Am Rev Respir Dis 1989;139:1179–1187.

47. Bates DV. Uptake of CO in health and emphysema. Clin Sci 1952;11:21–32.

48. Epler GR, Saber FA, Gaensler EA. Determination of severe impairment (disability) in interstitial lung disease. Am Rev Respir Dis 1980;121:647–659.

49. Nordenfelt I, Svensson G. The transfer factor (diffusing capacity) as a predictor of hypoxemia during exercise in restrictive and chronic obstructive pulmonary disease. Clin Physiol 1987;7:423–430.

50. Hyatt RE, Scanlon PD, Nakamura M. Interpretation of Pulmonary Function Tests: A Practical Guide, Second Edition. Lippincott Williams & Wilkins, Philadelphia, PA, 2003.

51. Cinkotai FF, Thomson ML. Diurnal variation in pulmonary diffusing capacity for carbon monoxide. J Appl Physiol 1966;21:539–542.

52. Frey TM, Crapo RO, Jensen RL, Elliott CG. Diurnal variation of the diffusing capacity of the lung: is it real? Am Rev Respir Dis 1987;136:1381–1384.

53. Sansores RH, Abboud RT, Kennell C, Haynes N. The effect of menstruation on the pulmonary carbon monoxide diffusing capacity. Am J Respir Crit Care Med 1995;151:381–384.

54. Peavy HH, Summer WR, Gurtner C. The effects of acute ethanol ingestion on pulmonary diffusing capacity. Chest 1980;77:488–492.

55. Frey TM, Crapo RO, Jensen RL, Elliott CG. Diurnal variation of the diffusing capacity of the lung: is it real? Am Rev Respir Dis 1987;136:1381–1384.

Chapter 4
Bronchial Challenge Testing

DEFINITIONS

Bronchial Challenge

- Is a test used to help in diagnosing or excluding bronchial asthma by provoking a bronchoconstriction response to a controlled external stimulus. The external stimulus varies according to the type of asthma. It could be a drug such as methacholine or a physical stimulus such as exercise or cold air.

Methacholine

- Is the most popular drug used in bronchial challenge*. Methacholine is an acetylcholine derivative that stimulates the cholinergic (muscarinic) receptors in the bronchial smooth muscle cells resulting in their contraction. This will cause bronchoconstriction at low methacholine concentrations in asthmatics.
- A significant bronchoconstrictive response is defined as a drop in FEV_1 by $\geq 20\%$ of its baseline value. The degree of airway reactivity is defined by the dose or concentration (PD_{20} or PC_{20}) of methacholine resulting in bronchoconstriction.

---

*This test is sometimes called *methacholine challenge test.*

A. Altalag et al., *Pulmonary Function Tests in Clinical Practice,*
DOI: 10.1007/978-1-84882-231-3_4, © Springer-Verlag London Limited 2009

PD_{20} or PC_{20}

- Stands for *provocative dose* or *provocative concentration*, respectively, that is, the dose or concentration of the drug at which a 20% decrease in FEV_1 occurs. This means that a drop of $\geq 20\%$ in FEV_1 is required for the provocative test to be positive. If the provocative test is positive, PD_{20} or PC_{20} is used to grade the severity of the provocative response.[1] The lower the PD_{20} or PC_{20} (i.e., the lower the concentration of methacholine in mg/ml), the more severe the responsiveness is.

BACKGROUND

- In asthmatics, the bronchial response to an allergen consists of two phases:
  - *Immediate response*, which occurs within few minutes of the exposure and is due to bronchial smooth muscle contraction (bronchospasm). This response can be blocked by bronchodilators or cromolyn sodium.
  - *Delayed response*, which occurs 6–12h following exposure and is due to airway inflammation. This can be blocked by steroids.
- Different allergens may produce either one or both responses. Methacholine produces only the immediate response but it is a good predictor of both responses caused by any allergen.
- Because methacholine responsiveness can be blocked by bronchodilators, the patient should be off these drugs to achieve the best results; Table 4.1.

TABLE 4.1. Minimum time interval for drugs that may influence methacholine test result

Inhaled Bronchodilators	
Short-acting agents (e.g., salbutamol, isoproterenol)[21, 38]	8h
Medium-acting agents (e.g., ipratropium)[17, 39]	24h
Long-acting agents (e.g., salmeterol, formoterol)[18, 20, 40]	48h
Long-acting oral theophyllines[41, 42]	48h
Cromolyn sodium[1]	8h
Leukotriene antagonists[1]	24h
Caffeine-containing foods[22]	Avoid on the study day
Inhaled or systemic steroids[1, 19]	No need to be stopped

TECHNIQUE

- The patient should be clinically stable, and the technician should be trained in how to deal with any unwanted response, such as severe bronchospasm or systemic reactions.[1] This test is done routinely in any standard pulmonary function laboratory or in specialized respiratory clinics and is generally safe.[8-15] Medical help should be readily available in rare case of a severe reaction though.
- The test and the possible side effects should be explained to the patient.
- The test is started by doing a baseline spirometry to record the initial FEV_1. If the spirometry reveals that the FEV_1 is less than 1L or <50% of predicted value, then the test should be abandoned because it is likely to cause trouble to the patient (very low baseline FEV_1).[2] The baseline spirometry tests need to be reproducible to allow comparison with later tests.
- After spirometry, the patient is nebulized with normal saline. Some patients are so hyperresponsive that saline can precipitate a bronchospastic reaction. These patients should not be tested with methacholine. The technician will report this observation for the interpreter.
- Methacholine starting dose or concentration is then selected according to different dosing protocols[†,1] (usually 2 ml of 1–2 mg/ml solution) and delivered to the patient via a nebulizer over 2min.[27-35] FEV_1 is then measured at 30s and 3min after nebulization.[1, 8, 16] To protect the PFT laboratory staff from exposure, nebulization is preferably performed in a negative pressure room.
- The dose of methacholine is then doubled and the test is repeated in a stepwise fashion until the patient reaches the maximum concentration of methacholine allowed (16mg/ml) or the test becomes positive. Table 4.2 lists indication for study termination.
- A short acting β_2-agonist (2–4 puffs of salbutamol through a spacing device) is then given to subjects who develop bronchoconstriction and the spirometry is repeated 15min after that. The results are plotted as a graph; Figure 4.1. The patient should be observed until he or she is clinically stable and FEV_1 is back to or near baseline.

---

†Two major dosing protocols are widely used: (1) the 2-min tidal breathing method (the method discussed in this chapter) and (2) the five-breath dosimeter method.[1]

TABLE 4.2. Indications for study termination

Achieving the maximum dose or concentration allowed without a
20% or greater drop in FEV_1

A positive test is achieved (drop in FEV_1 by ≥20% of baseline)

Patient becomes unstable clinically (dyspnea, wheezing, cough)

Patient develops systemic reaction (flushing, headache)

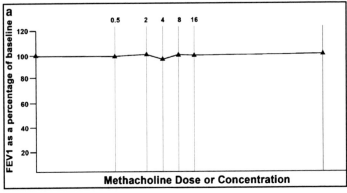

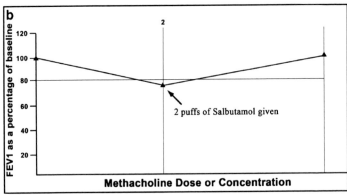

FIGURE 4.1. (a) A negative bronchial challenge test; the y-axis represents
the patient FEV_1 as a percentage of the baseline FEV_1 (before giving methacholine) and the x-axis represents the concentration of methacholine. The
maximum dose was reached without a significant reduction in FEV_1, indicating a negative test. (b) A positive bronchial challenge test, as 2 mg/ml of
methacholine resulted in a significant drop in FEV_1 indicating a positive
test. Two puffs of salbutamol resulted in restoration of FEV_1.

- Challenge testing can be done using other stimuli[1]:
  - Other drugs such as histamine
  - Exercise – in suspected exercise-induced asthma
  - Exposure to cold air – in cold air-induced asthma
  - Spirometry before and after work, in suspected occupational asthma.[‡]

INDICATIONS AND CONTRAINDICATIONS FOR BRONCHIAL CHALLENGE[1]

- The test is indicated when asthma is suspected but not obvious clinically or through spirometry as spirometry may be normal in stable asthmatics. Table 4.3 summarizes the major indications and contraindications for bronchial challenge test. In many laboratories a positive response to bronchodilator negates the need for a methacholine challenge test.

TABLE 4.3. Indications and contraindications for bronchial challenge

Indications for bronchial challenge
Unexplained dyspnea, cough, or episodic chest tightness
Unexplained dyspnea with exercise or cold-air exposure
A normal spirometry and bronchodilator response in a patient with a clinical picture suggestive of asthma
Mild airflow obstruction without a bronchodilator response
Absolute contraindications
Severe airflow limitation (FEV_1 <1 L or <50% predicted)[2]
A recent MI or CVA (within 3 months)
Arterial aneurysm especially if advanced
Hypertension (systolic >200 or diastolic >100 mmHg)
Relative contraindications
Moderate airflow limitation (FEV_1 <1.5 L or <60% predicted)[3, 4]
Clinical instability including a recent respiratory tract infection (test may be positive)
Inability to perform acceptable-quality spirometry
Pregnancy or nursing mothers
Current use of cholinesterase inhibitors (for myasthenia gravis)
Epilepsy

[‡] Or by exposure to workplace allergens thought to cause occupational asthma.

INTERPRETATION

- This test is very sensitive but non-specific. If negative, it almost excludes active asthma,[36, 37] except if the patient took a bronchodilator prior to the test. This means that almost all subjects with active asthma will have a positive test, but the test may be normal if asthma is in remission. A positive test can be seen in a variety of conditions, which are summarized in Table 4.4.[5–7] Therefore, a positive test should be reported as supportive of asthma, and a negative test makes asthma very unlikely.[1] Severe bronchial reactivity, however, may be considered diagnostic for bronchial asthma.
- Grading of severity of bronchial hyperresponsiveness based on PC_{20} is summarized in Table 4.5.[1]
- Figure 4.1 gives examples of a negative and a positive methacholine challenge test.

Table 4.4. Conditions associated with increase in bronchial reactivity[5–7]

Bronchial asthma
Allergic rhinitis
Sarcoidosis (up to 50% can have a positive test)
COPD
Cystic fibrosis
Recent respiratory tract infection[23–26]

Table 4.5. Grading of severity of bronchial hyperresponsiveness (based on PC_{20})[1]

Normal	PC_{20}>16mg/ml
Borderline	4–16
Mild	1–4
Moderate–severe	<1

References

1. American Thoracic Society. Guidelines for methacholine and exercise challenge testing – 1999. Am J Respir Crit Care Med 2000;161:309–329.
2. Martin RJ, Wanger JS, Irvin CG, Bartelson BB, Cherniack RM, the Asthma Clinical Research Network (ACRN). Methacholine challenge testing: safety of low starting FEV$_1$. Chest 1997;112:53–56.

3. Sterk PJ, Fabbri LM, Quanjer PH, Cockcroft DW, O'Byrne PM, Anderson SD, Juniper EF, Malo JL. Airway responsiveness: standardized challenge testing with pharmacological, physical and sensitizing stimuli in adults. Statement of the European Respiratory Society. Eur Respir J Suppl 1993;16:53–83.

4. Tashkin DP, Altose MD, Bleecker ER, Connett JE, Kanner RE, Lee WW, Wise R, the Lung Health Research Group. The Lung Health Study: airway responsiveness to inhaled methacholine in smokers with mild to moderate airflow limitation. Am Rev Respir Dis 1992;145:301–310.

5. Ramsdell JW, Nachtwey FJ, Moser KM. Bronchial hyperactivity in chronic obstructive bronchitis. Am Rev Respir Dis 1982;126(5):829–832.

6. Du Toit JI, Woolcock AJ, Salome CM, Sundrum R, Black JL. 1986. Characteristics of bronchial hyperresponsiveness in smokers with chronic air-flow limitation. Am Rev Respir Dis 134:498–501.

7. Yan K, Salome CM, Woolcock AJ. 1985. Prevalence and nature of bronchial hyperresponsiveness in subjects with chronic obstructive pulmonary disease. Am Rev Respir Dis 132:25–29.

8. Shapiro GG, Simon RA, for the American Academy of Allergy and Immunology Bronchoprovocation Committee. Bronchoprovocation committee report. J Allergy Clin Immunol 1992;89:775–778.

9. Martin RJ, Wanger JS, Irvin CG, Bartelson BB, Cherniack RM, the Asthma Clinical Research Network (ACRN). Methacholine challenge testing: safety of low starting FEV. Chest 1997;112:53–56.

10. Tashkin DP, Altose MD, Bleecker ER, Connett JE, Kanner RE, Lee WW, Wise R, the Lung Health Research Group. The Lung Health Study: airway responsiveness to inhaled methacholine in smokers with mild to moderate airflow limitation. Am Rev Respir Dis 1992;145:301–310.

11. Scott GC, Braun SR. A survey of the current use and methods of analysis of bronchoprovocational challenges. Chest 1991;100:322–328.

12. Weiss ST, Tager IB, Weiss JW, Munoz A, Speizer FE, Ingram RH. Airways responsiveness in a population sample of adults and children. Am Rev Respir Dis 1984;129:898–902.

13. Rijcken B, Schouten JP, Weiss ST, Speizer FE, van der Lende R. The relationship between airway responsiveness to histamine and pulmonary function level in a random population sample. Am Rev Respir Dis 1988;137:826–832.

14. Baake PS, Baste V, Gulsvik A. Bronchial responsiveness in a Norwegian community. Am Rev Respir Dis 1991;143:317–322.

15. Peat JK, Salome CM, Xuan W. On adjusting measurements of airway responsiveness for lung size and airway caliber. Am J Respir Crit Care Med 1996;154:870–875.

16. Lundgren R, Siiderberg M, Rosenhall L, Norman E. Case report: development of increased airway responsiveness in two nurses performing methacholine and histamine challenge tests. Allergy 1992;47:188–189.

17. Crimi N, Palermo F, Oliveri R, Polosa R, Settinieri I, Mistretta A. Protective effects of inhaled ipratropium bromide on bronchoconstriction

induced by adenosine and methacholine in asthma. Eur Respir J 1992;5:560–565.

18. Rabe KF, Jorres R, Nowak D, Behr N, Magnussen H. Comparison of the effects of salmeterol and formoterol on airway tone and responsiveness over 24 hours in bronchial asthma. Am Rev Respir Dis 1993;147:1436–1441.

19. Prieto L, Berto JM, Gutierrez V, Tornero C. Effect of inhaled budesonide on seasonal changes in sensitivity and maximal response to methacholine in pollen-sensitive asthmatic subjects. Eur Respir J 1994;7:1845–1851.

20. Cockcroft DW, Swystun VA, Bhagat R. Interaction of inhaled Bz agonist and inhaled corticosteroid on airway responsiveness to allergen and methacholine. Am J Respir Crit Care Med 1995;152:1485–1489.

21. Greenspon LW, Morrissey WL. Factors that contribute to inhibition of methacholine-induced bronchoconstriction. Am Rev Respir Dis 1986;133:735–739.

22. Henderson JC, O'Connell F, Fuller RW. Decrease of histamine induced bronchoconstriction by caffeine in mild asthma. Thorax 1993;48:824–826.

23. Cheung D, Dick EC, Timmers MC, deKlerk EPA, Spaan WJM, Sterk PJ. Rhinovirus inhalation causes long-lasting excessive airway narrowing in response to methacholine in asthmatic subjects in viva. Am J Respir Crit Care Med 1995;152:1490–1496.

24. Little JW, Hall WJ, Douglas RG, Mudholkar GS, Speers DM, Patel K. Airway hyperreactivity and peripheral airway dysfunction in influenza A infection. Am Rev Respir Dis 1978;118:295–303.

25. Annesi I, Oryszczyn M-P, Neukirch F, Oroven-Frija E, Korobaeff M, Kauffmann F. Relationship of upper airways disorders [rhinitis] to FEV, and bronchial hyperresponsiveness in an epidemiological study. Eur Respir J 1992;5:1104–1110.

26. Prieto JL, Gutierrez V, Berto JM, Camps B. Sensitivity and maximal response to methacholine in perennial and seasonal allergic rhinitis. Clin Exp Allergy 1996;26:61–67.

27. Juniper EF, Cockcroft DW, Hargreave FE. Tidal breathing method. In: Juniper EF, Cockcroft DW, Hargreave FE, eds. Histamine and Methacholine Inhalation Tests: Laboratory Procedure and Standardization, Second Edition. Astra Draco AB, Lund, Sweden, 1994.

28. Cockcroft DW, Killian DN, Mellon JJ, Hargreave FE. Bronchial reactivity to inhaled histamine: a method and clinical survey. Clin Allergy 1977;7:235–243.

29. Toelle BG, Peat JK, Salome CM, Crane J, McMillan D, Dermand J, D'Souza W, Woolcock AJ. Comparison of two epidemiological protocols for measuring airway responsiveness and allergic sensitivity in adults. Eur Respir J 1994;7:1798–1804.

30. Ryan G, Dolovich MB, Roberts RS, Frith PA, Juniper EF, Hargreave FE, Newhouse MT. Standardization of inhalation provocation tests:

two techniques of aerosol generation and inhalation compared. Am Rev Respir Dis 1981;123:195–199.

31. Beaupre A, Malo JL. Comparison of histamine bronchial challenges with the Wright nebulizer and the dosimeter. Clin Allergy 1979;9: 575–583.

32. Britton J, Mortagy A, Tattersfield AE. Histamine challenge testing: comparison of three methods. Thorax 1986;41:128–132.

33. Bennett JB, Davies RJ. A comparison of histamine and methacholine bronchial challenges using the DeVilbiss 646 nebulizer and the Rosenthal-French dosimeter. Br J Dis Chest 1987;81:252–259.

34. Knox AJ, Wisniewski A, Cooper S, Tattersfield AE. A comparison of the Yan and a dosimeter method for methacholine challenge in experienced and inexperienced subjects. Eur Respir J 1991;4:497–502.

35. Peat JK, Salome CM, Bauman A, Toelle BG, Wachinger SL, Woolcock AJ. Repeatability of histamine bronchial challenge and comparability with methacholine bronchial challenge in a population of Australian schoolchildren. Am Rev Respir Dis 1991;144:338–343.

36. Gilbert R, Auchincloss JH. Post-test probability of asthma following methacholine challenge. Chest 1990;97:562–565.

37. Cockcroft DW, Murdock KY, Berscheid BA, Gore BP. Sensitivity and specificity of histamine PC-20 determination in a random selection of young college students. I. Allergy Clin Immunol 1992;89:23–30.

38. Ahrens RC, Bonham AC, Maxwell GA, Weinberger MM. A method for comparing the peak intensity and duration of action of aerosolized bronchodilators using bronchoprovocation with methacholine. Am Rev Respir Dis 1984;129:903–906.

39. Wilson NM, Green S, Coe C, Barnes PJ. Duration of protection by oxitropium bromide against cholinergic challenge. Eur J Respir Dis 1987;71:455–458.

40. Derom EY, Pauwels RA, Van Der Straeten MEF. The effect of inhaled salmeterol on methacholine responsiveness in subjects with asthma up to 12 hours. J Allergy Clin Immunol 1902;89:811–815.

41. McWilliams BC, Menendez R, Kelley HW, Howick J. Effects of theophylline on inhaled methacholine and histamine in asthmatic children. Am Rev Respir Dis 1984;130:193–197.

42. Magnussen H, Reuss G, Jorres R. Theophylline has a doserelated effect on the airway response to inhaled histamine and methacholine in asthmatics. Am Rev Respir Dis 1987;136:1163–1167.

Chapter 5

Respiratory Muscle Function and Other Pulmonary Function Studies

RESPIRATORY MUSCLE FUNCTION

Maximal Respiratory Pressures

The two self-explanatory tests used to assess the respiratory pressures are the *maximal inspiratory pressure* (MIP)* and the *maximal expiratory pressure* (MEP).These pressures are generated by the respiratory muscles during a forceful inspiration and expiration, respectively.

Indications

- Assessment of respiratory muscle function:
  - In patients with known NMD
  - In patients with suspected early NMD (unexplained dyspnea or unexplained restrictive pattern in PFT)
- Particularly helpful when lung mechanics are abnormal, i.e., coexistent interstitial lung disease.

Technique

- To measure MIP, the patient is instructed to exhale fully (to RV) and then inhale against a closed valve as hard as possible. The resulting pressure should be sustained for 1 s. The test is repeated

---

*MIP and MEP are sometimes referred to as P_{Imax} and P_{Emax}, respectively.

A. Altalag et al., *Pulmonary Function Tests in Clinical Practice*,
DOI: 10.1007/978-1-84882-231-3_5, © Springer-Verlag London Limited 2009

for reproducibility and the highest reproducible pressure (i.e., within 20%) is reported.[2] Most laboratories use a flanged mouthpiece because it is easier to use as compared to the firmer rubber tube.[3,4] A small leak is introduced (a 2-mm hole in the tubing) to prevent glottic closure and use of the cheeks during MIP maneuver. For both MIP and MEP the maximum average pressure sustained for 1 s is recorded to avoid recording a brief peak, which is considered a pressure transient.

- To measure MEP, the patient inhales to TLC and then exhales against a closed valve as hard as possible. Similarly, the pressure has to be sustained for 1.5 s and the highest reproducible pressure is reported.

Interpretation

- The MIP is considered normal if it is below -70 cmH$_2$O and MEP above $+90$ cmH$_2$O in young adult males (lower values are reported in females and elderly).[†,5] Low MIP and MEP are seen in NMD even in early stages, when the physical weakness is not clinically apparent.[2] For causes of NMD, see Table 5.1.

TABLE 5.1. Causes of NMD

Neurogenic causes
Motor neuron disease or amyotrophic lateral sclerosis (ALS)
Guillain-barre syndrome
Poliomyelitis
Multiple sclerosis
High spinal cord injury (quadriplegia)
Phrenic nerve injury
Neuromuscular junction causes
Myasthenia gravis
Eaton–Lambert syndrome
Muscular causes
Muscular dystrophy
Myopathies (polymyositis, thyroid-related, inflammatory, lupus, steroid-induced, biochemical)
Malnutrition

---

†There is a wide range of normal values in the same age and sex; the normal values vary significantly with age and sex. For more details refer to the following references 2,3,7–18.

- Because the diaphragm is the major inspiratory muscle, in bilateral diaphragmatic paralysis, the MIP is usually low with a preserved MEP. On the other hand, in quadriparesis due to cord injury (below C3-5 where phrenic nerve originates), the MEP is low with a relatively preserved MIP, as the diaphragm is not affected.
- MIP can also be decreased in a poor-effort study and in patients with significant hyperinflation and air-trapping (like emphysema).[2] The degree of air-trapping and hyperinflation is directly proportional to the degree of impairment of the respiratory pressures. This effect is a result of the reduction in diaphragm muscle length that occurs when lung volume increases. Shorter length leads to low ability to shorten and produce a pressure. The same principle underlies the reason why MIP is measured at RV and MEP at TLC.
- MEP of <40 is predictive of an ineffective cough.[1, 6]

Limitations

- There is a wide range of normal results, making it sometimes difficult to separate normal from abnormal results.
- The test is effort dependent, and poor effort may mimic disease.

Sniff Tests

- Are designed to assess the strength of the diaphragm and the other inspiratory muscles. A sniff is a short, sharp voluntary inspiratory maneuver performed through one or both unoccluded nostrils. To be useful as a test of respiratory muscle strength, sniffs need to be maximal, which is relatively easy for most willing subjects, but may require some practice. Most subjects achieve reproducible values within 5–10 attempts.[2]
- Three sniff tests are available for clinical and research use:
  (a) *Sniff nasal pressure (sniff P_{nas})* is the least invasive among the other sniff tests and most practical in the clinical setting. It is measured by placing a plug in one nostril and measuring the pressure in the nose via a pressure catheter passed through the plug. Sniffing with the unoccluded nostril and with mouth closed will generate a negative pressure in the nose, which represents a reasonable approximation of the esophageal pressure (P_{es} – used to reflect intrathoracic pressure).[19, 20] A negative pressure of >60 cmH_2O excludes significant inspiratory muscle weakness.[21] In COPD, sniff P_{nas} tends to underestimate the esophageal pressure but

can complement MIP in excluding significant inspiratory muscle weakness.[22]

(b) *Sniff esophageal pressure (sniff P_{es})* is similarly measured by an esophageal balloon catheter system (a pressure sensing device on the end of a thin hollow tube) during maximal sniffs, and is indicated when the sniff P_{nas} is inconclusive. Sniff P_{es}, again, assesses the global inspiratory muscles strength including the diaphragm.[23] A negative pressure of >80 cmH$_2$O in men and >70 cmH$_2$O in women excludes significant inspiratory muscle weakness.[24]

(c) *Sniff transdiaphragmatic pressure (sniff P_{di})* measurement is performed by passing an esophageal and a gastric balloon and measuring the pressure difference on both sides of the diaphragm (transdiaphragmatic pressure) during maximal sniffs. Sniff P_{di} specifically measures diaphragmatic strength. A sniff P_{di} of >100 cmH$_2$O in men and >70 cmH$_2$O in women excludes significant diaphragmatic weakness.[24] A sniff P_{di} of <30 cmH$_2$O is associated with orthopnea, paradoxical abdominal motion, and a supine fall in VC, all of which are highly diagnostic for diaphragmatic paralysis.[25]

Transcutaneous Electrical Phrenic Nerve Stimulation

- Diaphragmatic function can be assessed nonvolitionally by stimulating the phrenic nerve(s), transcutaneously at FRC using an electrode placed over the skin at the posterior border of the sternocledomastoid.[2] This test is particularly useful in identifying muscle weakness when lack of effort is an issue, e.g., malingering. Supramaximal stimulation can be performed resulting in maximal diaphragmatic contraction that can be measured as a transdiaphragmatic pressure (twitch P_{di}) using gastric and esophageal balloons.

- One or both hemidiaphragms may be stimulated at once (single pulse). A resultant twitch P_{di} pressure of >10 cmH$_2$O (unilateral) or >20 cmH$_2$O (bilateral) excludes significant diaphragmatic weakness.[24]

- Although this test is effort-independent, the electrical stimulation can be uncomfortable and does not always produce a supramaximal stimulation, which can make it difficult to interpret subnormal results.

- Magnetic stimulation of phrenic nerve may be used instead of the electrical stimulation. Magnetic stimulation is less uncomfortable but is less widely used because of high equipment costs.[2, 24]

- The continuity of the phrenic nerve is assessed as the EMG of the diaphragm and is recorded using an esophageal electrode or, more commonly, a surface electrode placed in the seventh intercostal space at the midaxillary line (normal phrenic nerve conduction time is <9.5 ms).[‡,24] This test can substantiate diaphragmatic paralysis.

Cough Test

- Is used to assess the expiratory muscle strength because cough is a natural maneuver that can produce MEP. This pressure is measured using a gastric balloon catheter and is referred to as cough gastric pressure (cough P_{ga}). Patients with low MEP can have a normal cough P_{ga}, which indicates that this test may be more reliable than MEP but is more invasive at the same time.[2, 24] Peak cough flow rates are much less invasive and provide important information regarding airway clearance in patients suspected of having a weak cough.

Supine Spirometry

- Is indicated when diaphragmatic weakness is suspected. The FVC is significantly reduced in the supine position in such conditions because of elimination of gravity.
- A drop in FVC of <10% of the sitting value is considered normal.[26] Bilateral diaphragmatic paralysis is considered when FVC drops by >30% of the sitting value.[35]

Other Less Widely used Tests to Assess Respiratory Muscle Function

- Maximum mouth pressure
- Maximal static transdiaphragmatic pressure
- Abdominal muscle stimulation test
- Cough flow rates

OTHER PULMONARY FUNCTION STUDIES

Maximum Voluntary Ventilation (MVV)

- Is the maximum volume of air that can be breathed in and out over 1 min (liters/minute).

[‡]Bilateral tetanic stimulation can give maximal P_{di} but is uncomfortable and only used for research.

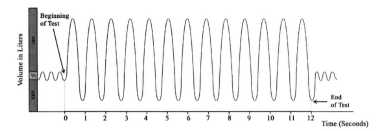

FIGURE 5.1. Measuring MVV in the laboratory. The test is done over 12 s and the result is extrapolated to 60 s by multiplying by 5.

- It is measured in the laboratory by asking the patient to breathe as fast and as hard as possible for 12 s, then the result is extrapolated to 1 min by multiplying that by 5; see Figure 5.1.
- MVV correlates very well with FEV_1, and it can also be estimated by multiplying the patient's FEV_1 by 40 (some prefer 35).[27–32] If the measured MVV is significantly lower than the calculated one, then this may suggest a poor effort.
- MVV is a very nonspecific test and is usually reduced with any pulmonary disorder (obstructive or restrictive disorders including NMD), being more significantly lower in obstructive disorders. MVV is also reduced in poor effort test and in cardiac disease.
- MVV has, however, an important role in assessing the ventilatory function during exercise, as it correlates well with the maximal exercise capacity (see Chapter 9 for details).

Airway Resistance (R_{AW}) and Conductance (G_{AW})

- R_{AW} (L/s/cmH$_2$O) is the amount of pressure (alveolar pressure over the mouth pressure or the transpulmonary pressure) required to generate a given airflow, while G_{AW} (cmH$_2$O/L/s) is the reciprocal of that, i.e., the amount of airflow generated by a given alveolar pressure.
- These tests are not effort-dependent and are used in patients with suspected obstructive disorders who cannot produce good effort in spirometry.[33, 34] They are, however, prone to measurement and calculation errors, which limit their use.
- Their measurement involves measuring the mouth and alveolar pressures in the body box at FRC, while also measuring the lung volumes. The flow, measured at the mouth, divided by the difference between alveolar and mouth pressures represents R_{AW}. The reciprocal of that is G_{AW}. Because the lung volume at which

the flow is measured will influence the airway resistance, the results are corrected to that lung volume to generate the *specific airway resistance* and *conductance* (SR_{AW}, SG_{AW}).

- An increased R_{AW} is likely to be due to an obstructive disorder.

Lung Compliance (C_L)

- Is the change in lung volume for a given change in pressure or simply, the ability of the lung to expand. It is measured by simultaneous measurements of the lung volume and the elastic recoil pressure by an esophageal balloon (P_{es}).
- C_L can be expressed in two ways, static or dynamic lung compliance (C_{Lstat} and C_{Ldyn}):
  (a) C_{Lstat} is calculated by measuring the pressure when there is no flow at two different lung volumes. It is decreased in lung fibrosis (decreased ability of the lung to expand) and increased in emphysema.
  (b) C_{Ldyn} is measured during tidal breathing (V_T) by continuously measuring pressure and volume (C_{Ldyn} is represented as $\Delta P/\Delta V$). C_{Ldyn} is lower than C_{Lstat} in patients with airway obstruction. In these patients, C_{Ldyn} decreases further as frequency of breathing increases.[24, §]
- *Total thoracic compliance* is the compliance of both the lungs and chest wall together. It can only be reliably measured in ventilated and paralyzed patients where activity of the chest wall muscles is eliminated. It is decreased in disease of either the chest wall (ankylosing spondylitis) or the lungs (acute respiratory distress syndrome, ARDS).

Forced Oscillation Technique (Oscillometry)

- Is the determination of the total pulmonary resistance by imposing known variations in flow at the mouth and measuring the resultant pressure changes.
- Because it measures the total resistance, it is hard to separate the upper from the lower airway resistance, which limits its clinical usefulness.
- Its main use is in children who cannot generally perform spirometric maneuvers.

---

§ This reduction is caused by the effect of the increasing frequency of breathing on the lung units that are recruited. As the frequency of breathing increases, the lung units with more rapid frequency response, i.e., shorter time constant, are recruited and these units are less compliant.

References

1. Hyatt RE, Scanlon PD, Nakamura M. Interpretation of Pulmonary Function Tests: A Practical Guide, 2nd Edition. Lippincott Williams & Wilkins, Philadelphia, PA, 2003.

2. Green M, Road J, Sieck GC, Similowski T. ATS/ERS statement on respiratory muscle testing: tests of respiratory muscle strength. Am J Respir Crit Care Med 2002;166:518–624.

3. Black L, Hyatt R. Maximal respiratory pressures: normal values and relationship to age and sex. Am Rev Respir Dis 1969;99:696–702.

4. Koulouris N, Mulvey DA, Laroche CM, Green M, Moxham J. Comparison of two different mouthpieces for the measurement of PImax and PEmax in normal and weak subjects. Eur Respir J 1988;1:863–867.

5. Enright PL, Kronmal RA, Manolio TA, Schenker MB, Hyatt RE. Respiratory muscle strength in the elderly: correlates and reference values. Am J Respir Crit Care Med 1994;149:430–438.

6. Hancox B, Whyte K. Pocket Guide to Lung Function Tests, 1st Edition. McGraw-Hill, Sydney, 2001.

7. Hamnegard CH, Wragg SD, Kyroussis D, Mills GH, Polkey MI, Moran J, Road JD, Bake B, Green M, Moxham J. Diaphragm fatigue following maximal ventilation in man. Eur Respir J 1996;9:241–247.

8. Mador JM, Rodis A, Diaz J. Diaphragmatic fatigue following voluntary hyperpnea. Am J Respir Crit Care Med 1996;154:63–67.

9. Polkey MI, Kyroussis D, Hamnegard CH, Mills GH, Hughes PD, Green M, Moxham J. Diaphragm performance during maximal voluntary ventilation in chronic obstructive pulmonary disease. Am J Respir Crit Care Med 1997;155:642–648.

10. Fitting JW, Bradley TD, Easton PA, Lincoln MJ, Goldman MD, Grassino A. Dissociation between diaphragmatic and rib cage muscle fatigue. J Appl Physiol 1988;64:959–965.

11. Hershenson MB, Kikuchi Y, Tzelepis GE, McCool D. Preferential fatigue of the rib cage muscles during inspiratory resistive loaded ventilation. J Appl Physiol 1997;66:750–754.

12. Roussos C, Gross D, Macklem PT. Fatigue of inspiratory muscles and their synergic behavior. J Appl Physiol 1979;46:897–904.

13. Nickerson BG, Keens TG. Measuring ventilatory muscle endurance in humans as sustainable inspiratory pressure. J Appl Physiol 1982;52: 768–772.

14. Clanton TL, Dixon GF, Drake J, Gadek JE. Effects of swim training on lung volumes and inspiratory muscle conditioning. J Appl Physiol 1987;62:39–46.

15. Clanton TL, Dixon G, Drake J, Gadek JE. Inspiratory muscle conditioning using a threshold loading device. Chest 1985;87:62–66.

16. Eastwood PR, Hillman DR. A threshold loading device for testing of inspiratory muscle performance. Eur Respir J 1995;8:463–466.

17. Martyn JB, Moreno RH, Pare PD, Pardy RL. Measurement of inspiratory muscle performance with incremental threshold loading. Am Rev Respir Dis 1987;135:919–923.

18. Belman MJ, Scott GT, Lewis MI. Resistive breathing training in patients with chronic obstructive pulmonary disease. Chest 1986;90:662–669.

19. Clanton TL, Ameredes BT. Fatigue of the inspiratory muscle pump in humans: an isoflow approach. J Appl Physiol 1988;64:1693–1699.

20. Mador MJ, Rodis A, Magalang UJ, Ameen K. Comparison of cervical magnetic and transcutaneous phrenic nerve stimulation before and after threshold loading. Am J Respir Crit Care Med 1996;154:448–453.

21. Heritier F, Rahm F, Pasche P, Fitting J-W. Sniff nasal pressure. Anon ivasive assessment of inspiratory muscle strength. Am J Respir Crit Care Med 1994;150:1678–1683.

22. Bellemare F, Grassino A. Evaluation of human diaphragm fatigue. J Appl Physiol 1982;53:1196–1206.

23. Laaroche CM, Mier AK, Moxham J, Green M. The value of sniff esophageal pressure in the assessment of global inspiratory muscle strength. Am Rev Respir Dis 1988;598–603.

24. Hughes JMB, Pride NB. Lung Function Tests, Physiological Principles and Clinical Applications, First Edition. W. B. Saunders, Philadelphia, 1999.

25. Mier A, Brophy C, Moxham H, Green M. Assessment of diaphragm weakness. Am Rev Respir Dis 1988;137:877–883.

26. Allen SM, Hunt B, Green M. Fall in vital capacity with posture. Br J Dis Chest 1995;79:267–271.

27. Punzal PA, Ries AL, Kaplan RM, Prewitt LM. Maximum intensity exercise training in patients with chronic obstructive pulmonary disease. Chest 1991;100:618–623.

28. Franciosa JA, Park M, Levine TB. Lack of correlation between exercise capacity and indexes of resting left ventricular performance in heart failure. Am J Cardiol 1981;47:33–39.

29. Weber KT, Janicki JS. Cardiopulmonary exercise testing: physiologic principles and clinical applications. W. B. Saunders, Philadelphia, 1986.

30. Szlachcic J, Massie BM, Kramer BL, Topic N, Tubau J. Correlates and prognostic implication of exercise capacity in chronic congestive heart failure. Am J Cardiol 1985;55:1037–1042.

31. Dillard TA, Piantadosi S, Rajagopal KR. Prediction of ventilation at maximal exercise in chronic air-flow obstruction. Am Rev Respir Dis 1985;132:230–235.

32. Dillard TA, Hnatiuk OW, McCumber TR. Maximum voluntary ventilation: spirometric determinants in chronic obstructive pulmonary disease patients and normal subjects. Am Rev Respir Dis 1993;147:870–875.

33. Pellegrino R, Viegi G, Enright P, et al. Interpretative strategies for lung function tests. Eur Respir J 2005;26:948–968.

34. Pride NB, Macklem PT. Lung mechanics in disease. In: Macklem PT, Mead J, eds. Handbook of Physiology. The Respiratory System. Mechanics of Breathing. Section 3, Vol. III, Part 2. American Physiological Society, Bethesda, MD. 1986;659–692.

35. Green M. Respiratory muscle testing. Bull Eur Physiol Respir 1984;20:433–436.

Chapter 6
Approach to PFT Interpretation

APPROACH OUTLINE

1. Review of clinical history provided, patient's demographics, and technician's comments
2. Examine the volume–time curve:
   - (a) Technical quality of the curve
   - (b) Size and shape
   - (c) Components
   - (d) Postbronchodilator curve
3. Examine the flow–volume curve/loop:
   - (a) Technical quality of the curve
   - (b) Size and shape
   - (c) Components
   - (d) Location
   - (e) Its relation to the tidal FV loop
   - (f) Postbronchodilator curve
4. Spirometry:
   - (a) Examine FVC, FEV_1, and FEV_1/FVC ratio.
   - (b) Examine the postbronchodilator value of FVC, FEV_1, and FEV_1/FVC ratio.
   - (c) Examine MMEF and FEFs.
   - (d) Examine the rest of the spirometry.
   - (e) Consider some special situations.
5. Lung volumes:
   - (a) Examine TLC, RV, and RV/TLC ratio.
   - (b) Examine the rest of the lung volumes (FRC, ERV, IC).
   - (c) Consider some special situations.

A. Altalag et al., *Pulmonary Function Tests in Clinical Practice*,
DOI: 10.1007/978-1-84882-231-3_6, © Springer-Verlag London Limited 2009

TABLE 6.1. Approach to PFT interpretation

Approach outline
  Review: clinical history provided, patient's demographics, and technician's
    comments
  Examine the volume–time curve
  Examine the flow–volume curve/loop, if available
  Examine the spirometry
  Examine the lung volumes
  Examine the gas transfer study
  Examine any additional test provided
  Compare the current study with previous ones, if available
**Reaching a useful conclusion (based on spiromerty and lung
  volume study)**
  Both are obstructive
  Both are restrictive
  Both are normal
  One is restrictive and the other is obstructive
  One is normal and the other is abnormal

6. Gas transfer study:
   (a) Examine DL_{CO} and DL_{CO}/V_A ratio.
   (b) Examine DL_{CO}/Hgb correction.
   (c) Examine the rest of the variables.
7. Examine any additional test provided:
   (a) Methacholine challenge
   (b) Maximum respiratory pressures
   (c) Supine spirometry
   (d) MVV, ABG, and other tests provided
8. Compare the current study with previous ones, if available.

See also Table 6.1. The following is an abbreviated version of what
we have reviewed in the previous chapters.

REVIEW THE CLINICAL HISTORY PROVIDED, PATIENT'S
DEMOGRAPHICS, AND TECHNICIAN'S COMMENTS

- The *clinical data* provided in the requisition form are important to
  direct the interpreter's attention as well as the final report. Clinical
  data are extremely useful in helping to form your conclusion.
- The *patient's demographics* also provide useful information, e.g.,
  the patient's weight (obesity can lead to a restrictive pattern).
- *Technicians' comments* provide information about the quality
  of the study, consistency with the ATS guidelines, and patient's
  effort. Technicians sometimes comment about the patient's condition, for example, the presence of kyphoscoliosis, wheezing,

or stridor while testing. This information may not be provided in the clinical data.

APPROACH TO VOLUME–TIME (VT) CURVE

- Examine the VT curve by observing:
  - *The duration of the curve* should be at least 6 s to meet the ATS criteria, and in the laboratory this is usually achievable.
  - *The size and shape of the curve* compared with the predicted curve:
    - (a) In obstructive disorder: the curve is less steep than the predicted curve.
    - (b) In restrictive disorder: the curve has a normal shape but is smaller than the predicted curve.
  - *The components of the curve* help to distinguish restrictive from obstructive abnormalities:
    - (a) FVC (the height of the curve)
    - (b) FEV_1 (the volume corresponding to 1 s)
    - (c) $FEF_{25,50,75,25-75}$ (extracted from the curve's slope)
  - *Post bronchodilator curve, if applicable*
    - (a) In patients with a suspected obstructive disorder, a post bronchodilator curve is also done (usually red in color). Improvement in the shape and slope of this curve compared to the original may indicate a response to bronchodilators. Comparing the heights (FVC) and the volume corresponding to 1 second (FEV_1) in both curves may help judging the response to bronchodilators more accurately; Figure 1.16.

APPROACH TO THE FLOW–VOLUME (FV) CURVE/LOOP

- *Assess the technical quality of the study based on FV curve*:
  - A good curve quality should have the following; Figure 1.11a[1, 2]:
    - (a) Good start (rapid climb to PEF, which should be sharp and rounded)
    - (b) Smooth curve free from artifacts (mainly in the 1st second)
    - (c) Good end (slight upward concavity at the end of the curve)
  - The lack of any of these criteria affects the study quality. Therefore, the results should then be interpreted with caution. The technician's comments address the patient's technique (if poor) and the study acceptability and reproducibility (which are impaired with a poor technique).
  - A morphologically poor start of the study should not prompt you to reject the study right away, as the same curve may be seen in NMD and in children; Figure 6.1f.

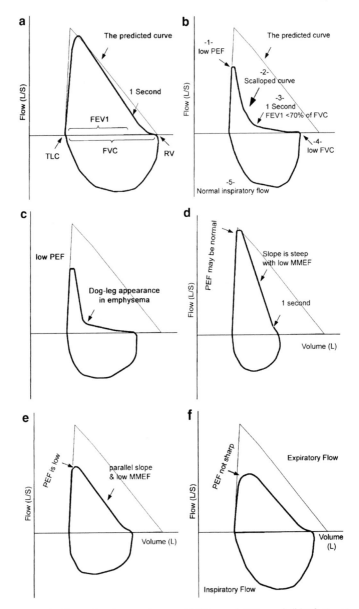

FIGURE 6.1. Normal and most abnormal FV loops: (**a**) Normal. (**b**) Obstructive loop. (**c**) Dog-leg obstructive curve, typical for emphysema. (**d**) Parenchymal restriction with a *witch's hat* appearance. (**e**) Chest wall restriction (consider racial variations). (**f**) NMD or poor initial effort (can also be seen in children). (**g**) Variable intrathoracic upper airway obstruction. (**h**) Variable extrathoracic upper airway obstruction. (**i**) Fixed upper airway obstruction.

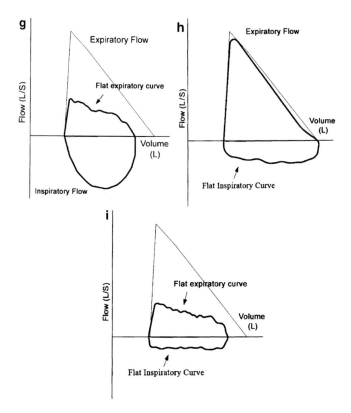

FIGURE 6.1. (continued)

- *Examine the size and shape of the FV curve/loop*:
  - The size and shape of the curve (after excluding poor quality curves) should fit one of the following; Figure 6.1:
    - (a) *Normal size and shape*; Figure 6.1a: indicates a normal study, including the normal variants such as the "knee" variant; Figure 1.22.
    - (b) *Small and concave or scooped*: suggests obstructive disorder; Figure 6.1b, c.
    - (c) *Small and steep slope* with a *witch's hat* shape: suggests parenchymal restriction; Figure 6.1d.
    - (d) *Small and parallel slope to the predicted curve*: is seen in chest wall restriction (musculoskeletal disease, diaphragmatic distention, and obesity) or normal patients with small lungs – racial variations; Figure 6.1e.

(e) *Small and convex shape* (mimicking poor start, i.e., delayed and decreased PEF, which is not sharp): is seen in a study with a poor effort, in NMD, and in children; Figure 6.1f.

(f) *Small and flat* (suggests central airway obstruction):
   * Only the expiratory component is flat (variable intrathoracic obstruction); Figure 6.1g.
   * Only the inspiratory component is flat (variable extrathoracic obstruction); Figure 6.1h.
   * Both components are flat (fixed obstruction); Figure 6.1i.

– This step is important in making a quick impression about the underlying disorder. This impression is usually correct.

• *Examine the components of the curve*:
   – *Height* (PEF) *and slope* (FEF_{25-75}) – if low, this may suggest an obstructive disorder.
   – *Width* (FVC) – if smaller than the predicted curve, suggests restrictive (mainly) or obstructive defect (to a lesser extent).
   – *The 1st second mark* (FEV_1) – check how it compares to the whole width of the curve (FVC) to visually estimate the FEV_1/FVC ratio. If low, it suggests obstruction; Figure 6.1b.

• *Examine the location of the curve compared to the predicted*:
   – This is only possible if spirometry is done in the body box while measuring lung volumes. If so, then we can apply the following; Figure 2.7:
   (a) If the curve runs along the predicted one, then TLC and RV are normal.
   (b) If the curve is shifted to the right (↓TLC, ↓RV), it suggests a restrictive defect (remember: shift to the right → restriction).
   (c) If the curve is shifted to the left (↑TLC, ↑RV), it suggests obstruction (If, in addition, FVC is ↓, then RV/TLC ratio should be ↑, supporting obstruction; think about that for a minute!).

• *Examine postbronchodilator curve, if applicable.*
   – As mentioned earlier, a prebronchodilator curve is colored in blue, while the postcurve is in red.
   – Quickly examine the technical quality of the red curve.
   – Then examine its shape, size, and location compared with the blue curve. If the red curve shows improvement in the shape, size, and/or location compared with the blue curve, it indicates a response to bronchodilators, which may be significant; Figure 1.15.

APPROACH TO SPIROMETRY

- *Examine FVC, FEV$_1$, and FEV$_1$/FVC ratio:*
  - There are four possibilities:
    (a) Normal – when all are normal.
    (b) Clearly obstructive – defined by a $\downarrow$ FEV$_1$/FVC ratio (FEV$_1$ is usually $\downarrow$ and FVC is relatively preserved; FEV$_1$ level (% pred.) determines severity; Table 1.4).
    (c) Possibly restrictive – with $\downarrow$ FVC and a normal or $\uparrow$ FEV$_1$/FVC ratio (confirm the restrictive nature of the disorder by measuring TLC, which should be low; if TLC is not done, FVC is used to grade severity; Table 1.4). Remember that spirometry with a poor effort may look restrictive.
    (d) Combined obstructive and restrictive disorder – may be suggested if the reduction in FVC is out of proportion to the reduction in the FEV$_1$/FVC ratio (e.g., the FEV$_1$/FVC ratio is 65% and FVC is only 40% pred.).[3] A normal FVC, however, rules out restriction.[4, 5] To be definite about the presence of a combined disorder, the lung volumes need to be examined.
- *Examine the postbronchodilator value of FVC, FEV$_1$, and FEV$_1$/ FVC ratio, if available.*
  - The response to bronchodilators can be as follows[6, 7]:
    (a) Significant response – 12% and 200 ml $\uparrow$ in FEV$_1$ or FVC.
    (b) Insignificant or no response – if it is less than that.
- *Examine FEF$_{25,50,75,25-75}$*
  - These flows usually follow the FEV$_1$. Therefore, if low, they suggest obstruction but can be low in restrictive disorders and upper airway obstruction. This defect is not specific for small airways disease.[6, 8]
- *Have a quick look at the rest of the spirometry:*
  - PEF decreases with the following:
    (a) Poor effort (as it is effort dependent)
    (b) Obstruction (mainly)
    (c) May decrease with restriction (such as NMD); it is usually preserved in parenchymal restriction.
  - PIF and FIF$_{50}$ – drop with poor effort or with variable extrathoracic obstruction (do not worry about this, as it will be obvious in FV loop, if available).
  - FET – helps knowing the appropriate duration of exhalation (should be ≥ 6 s). If excessively prolonged, it may suggest a mild airway obstruction.

- *Special situations*
  - Isolated reduction in MMEF and FEFs indicates airflow limitation at low lung volumes.[6, 8–11] Lung volume study may be of help.
  - An isolated significant response to bronchodilators with normal flows at baseline strongly suggests bronchial asthma.[6]

APPROACH TO LUNG VOLUME STUDY

- *Examine TLC, RV, and RV/TLC ratio* (these are the most important lung volume variables):
  - They usually change in the same direction, i.e., the direction of obstruction or restriction. The following are the possibilities:
  - (a) Normal, when all are normal.
  - (b) High volumes, suggesting obstruction; remember:
    - * ↑ TLC usually indicates hyperinflation (hyperinflation is more accurately defined by ↑ FRC).
    - * ↑ RV indicates air trapping.
    - * ↑ RV/TLC ratio reflects the degree of air trapping.[6]
  - (c) Low in restrictive disorders (↓TLC is essential to make a confident diagnosis of restriction[6]; TLC should be used to grade severity, if available; Table 1.4).
- *Examine the rest of the lung volumes (FRC, ERV, IC)*:
  - They usually follow the TLC and RV, so they are high in obstructive and low in restrictive disorders.
- *Special situations*:
  - Isolated reduction in ERV indicates obesity, check the patient's weight.
  - When the lung volumes are incompatible with spirometry, consider combined disorders; see next sections.

APPROACH TO GAS TRANSFER STUDY

- *Examine DL_{CO} and DL_{CO}/V_A ratio*:
  - For simplicity, consider four possibilities:
  - (a) Both are normal – this indicates that there is no gas-exchange abnormality.
  - (b) Both are high – seen in a variety of pulmonary and systemic disorders, review Table 3.3.
  - (c) DL_{CO}/V_A is low (regardless of the value of DL_{CO}) – this indicates a gas-exchange abnormality. Remember the causes of low DL_{CO} (Table 3.3) and consider the most important ones:
    - * Parenchymal lung disease

* Pulmonary vascular disease
* Anemia

(d) DL_{CO} is low with a normal or high DL_{CO}/V_A (i.e., it normalizes if corrected to V_A as the loss in V_A is the predominant abnormality) – unfortunately, you cannot conclude much from this. Consider the following:

* This could be an extraparenchymal disease (loss of alveolar spaces) such as lung resection or chest wall restriction (e.g., NMD).[12]
* Remember that gas-exchange abnormality like lung fibrosis cannot be excluded.
* Normal subjects who fail to take a deep enough breath or long enough breath-hold can show similar abnormalities; see next.

- *Examine DL_{CO}/Hgb correction, if Hgb is available*:[13–17]
  - If a low DL_{CO} corrects to normal, it indicates that anemia is responsible for the reduction in DL_{CO}.
  - If it does not correct to normal, then a gas-exchange abnormality rather than anemia is responsible.

- *Examine the rest of the variables*:
  - V_A should roughly equal TLC and is usually less than TLC. In an obstructive disorder, the difference between the two increases and roughly estimates the volume of the poorly ventilated air spaces; see also Table 6.2.
  - BHT and IVC help in determining the accuracy of DL_{CO} study:
    (a) BHT should equal 10 s. If less, DL_{CO} is underestimated and vice versa.
    (b) IVC should be at least 85% of the patient's VC. If less, DL_{CO} is underestimated and vice versa.[1]

TABLE 6.2. Methods to identify the presence of air trapping and estimate its volume

From spirometry: a significant difference between SVC and FVC indicates air trapping (SVC being larger than FVC).
From lung volume study: a high RV indicates air trapping; the difference between the measured and the predicted RV roughly estimates the volume of the trapped air.
From gas transfer study: a significantly higher TLC compared with V_A indicates air trapping.
N_2 *washout or gas dilution methods vs. plethysmography*: if TLC is estimated with plethysmography and either N_2 washout or gas dilution methods, then the difference between the two TLC measurements can estimate the volume of trapped air.

REACHING A USEFUL CONCLUSION

Combining spirometry, lung volumes and DL_{CO} measurements helps reach an accurate conclusion. Start by determining whether spirometry and lung volumes support the same diagnosis:

If both (spirometry and lung volumes) support an obstructive defect:

- The final diagnosis is then a *pure obstructive disorder.*
- You will need *then* to differentiate between the two major obstructive disorders – asthma and emphysema:
    - *FV curve*: a "dog-leg" appearance is characteristic for emphysema.[18]
    - *Spirometry*: a significant bronchodilator response is suggestive of asthma.
    - *Lung volume study*:
      (a) TLC is usually normal in asthma and ↑ in emphysema.
      (b) RV/TLC ratio is increased in emphysema and in asthma.[19, 20]
    - *DL_{CO}*: ↓ in emphysema and normal or ↑ in asthma.[21–26]
    - If you can estimate the degree of *air trapping*, see Table 6.2: it is much higher in emphysema than in asthma.
    - *Bronchial challenge*: is more likely to be positive in asthma than in emphysema.
- Remember that other obstructive disorders (such as bronchiectasis, obstructive bronchiolitis, and chronic bronchitis) could be responsible.

Both support a restrictive defect:

- The final diagnosis is then a *pure restrictive disorder.*
- The two major groups of disorder involved are as follows:
    - Parenchymal restriction, like ILD
    - Chest wall restriction (NMD, MSD, diaphragmatic paralysis and morbid obesity)
- The following helps for the distinction:
    - *FV curve*:
      (a) A small curve with a steep slope suggests a parenchymal restriction.
      (b) A small curve with a parallel slope to the predicted curve suggests a chest wall restriction other than NMD.
      (c) A convex curve (Figure 6.1f) suggests NMD or poor effort study.

– *Lung volumes*:

(a) Although the TLC is $\downarrow$ in both disorders, RV is usually normal or $\uparrow$ in chest wall restriction and $\downarrow$ in parenchymal restriction. The RV/TLC ratio is invariably $\uparrow$ in chest wall restriction (it is mostly normal with parenchymal restriction).[27]

(b) The degree of the reduction in FVC compared with TLC:
* If FVC and TLC are proportionally reduced, then this supports parenchymal restriction.
* If the reduction in FVC is out of proportion to the reduction in TLC (i.e., TLC is relatively preserved), this supports chest wall restriction.

– DL_{CO}[12]

(a) If low (DL_{CO}/V_A) – it supports parenchymal restriction.

(b) If normal (DL_{CO} and DL_{CO}/V_A) – it supports chest wall restriction

(c) If DL_{CO} is $\downarrow$ but DL_{CO}/V_A is normal or high – it supports chest wall restriction but cannot exclude a parenchymal restriction.

• To differentiate the types of chest wall restriction:

– Obesity:

(a) You can calculate the BMI; a BMI of >35 is compatible with obesity causing a restrictive pattern.

(b) ERV is usually very low in obesity

(c) Usually normal MIP and MEP.

– MSD (such as kyphoscoliosis):

(a) Normal or reduced[28] MIP and MEP (not such a large reduction as seen in NMD).

(b) Usually the history provided is suggestive of MSD.

– NMD (such as ALS)

(a) FV curve is usually convex in shape.

(b) MIP and MEP are $\downarrow$.[28]

– Diaphragmatic paralysis

(a) MIP is $\downarrow$ with a normal MEP (normal expiratory muscles).

(b) FVC is markedly reduced in supine position (drops by >30% from sitting FVC).[29]

(c) Other tests (transdiaphragmatic pressure is reduced).

If both are normal:

• Consider the *isolated abnormalities* before reporting the study as normal:

– *An isolated reduction of MMEF and FEFs*: indicates a non-specific airflow limitation at low lung volumes, as discussed.[6, 8–11]

- *Isolated reduction in ERV*: is usually associated with obesity.
- *Isolated reduction in DL_{CO}/V_A*: indicates a gas exchange abnormality. So, consider early parenchymal lung disease (such as emphysema or ILD), pulmonary vascular disease, or anemia.[12] An isolated reduction in DL_{CO} with a normal DL_{CO}/V_A should be reported as abnormal and similar causes explored.
- *Isolated significant response to bronchodilators* (with a normal prebronchodilator study): strongly suggests an obstructive defect[6] (bronchial asthma).

If the results of spirometry and lung volumes are opposite to each other:

- An obstructive spirometry ($\downarrow$ FEV_1/FVC ratio) with low lung volumes ($\downarrow$ TLC):
  - The two *major* possibilities are as follows:
    (a) A combined disorder.[3, 6]
    (b) An obstructive disorder with pulmonary resection (history may help).

- A restrictive spirometry with high lung volumes:
  - May represent a combined abnormality.
  - An obstructive disorder with severe air trapping or poor effort spirometry should be considered.[6]

If one study (spirometry or lung volume study) is normal and the other is abnormal:

- *Normal spirometry with abnormal lung volume study*
  - *Normal spirometry with low lung volumes*:
    (a) This is uncommon, and may represent a lab error as normal VC from spirometry excludes the restrictive abnormality suggested by low lung volumes.[3, 4]
  - *Normal spirometry with high lung volumes*:
    (a) Obstructive disorder:
      * Emphysema with minimal airway disease.
      * Mild asthma (if TLC is normal and RV is increased)[27]
    (b) Another possibility is acromegaly; a normal RV/TLC ratio is more likely with acromegaly than with obstruction. Another clue is $\uparrow$ FVC.[27] Patients with large lungs, e.g., swimmer may have similar values.

- *Normal lung volume study with abnormal spirometry*
  - *Normal lung volumes with an obstructive spirometry*:
    (a) A combined disorder

(b) Obstructive disorder with pulmonary resection (review the history)

(c) Pure obstructive disorder (e.g., bronchial asthma without air trapping)

- *Normal lung volumes with a restrictive spirometry*:

(a) Pure lung restriction is excluded because of a normal TLC. Four possibilities could be considered:

  * Poor effort (examine the FV curve morphology and review technician's comments)

  * Mild obstructive disorder, e.g., mild asthma, sometimes called pseudorestriction (grade according to FEV_1)[30, 31]; the following tests may be supportive:

    (1) ↑ Airway resistance

    (2) Significant bronchodilator response

    (3) Positive bronchial challenge

  * If *not* a poor effort study and there is no evidence of obstruction, report it as *non-specific ventilatory limitation*, which simply means, we do not know![27]

  * *Consider* a mild combined disorder.

References

1. Miller MR, Hankinson J, Brusasco V, et al. Standardisation of spirometry. Eur Respir J 2005;26:319–338.

2. American Thoracic Society. Standardization of spirometry, 1994 update. Am J Respir Crit Care Med 1995;152:1107–1136.

3. Dykstra BJ, Scanlon PD, Kester MM, Beck KC, Enright PL. Lung volumes in 4774 patients with obstructive lung disease. Chest 1999;115:68–74.

4. Aaron SD, Dales RE, Cardinal P. How accurate is spirometry at predicting restrictive impairment. Chest 1999;115:869–873.

5. Glady CA, Aaron SD, Lunau M, Clinch J, Dales RE. A spirometry-based algorithm to direct lung function testing in the pulmonary function laboratory. Chest 2003;123:1939–1946.

6. Pellegrino R, Viegi G, Enright P, et al. Interpretative strategies for lung function tests. Eur Respir J 2005;26:948–968.

7. Cerveri I, Pellegrino R, Dore R, et al. Mechanisms for isolated volume response to a bronchodilator in patients with COPD. J Appl Physiol 2000;88:1989–1995.

8. Flenley DC. Chronic obstructive pulmonary disease. Dis Mon 1988;34:537–599.

9. Bates DV. Respiratory Function in Disease, Third Edition. WB Saunders, Philadelphia, PA, 1989.

10. Wilson AF, ed. Pulmonary Function Testing, Indications and Interpretations. Grune & Stratton, Orlando, FL, 1985.

11. Pride NB, Macklem PT. Lung mechanics in disease. In: Macklem PT, Mead J, eds. Handbook of Physiology. The Respiratory System. Mechanics of Breathing. Section 3, Vol. III, Part 2. American Physiological Society, Bethesda, MD, 1986;659–692.

12. MacIntyre N, Crapo RO, Viegi G, et al. Standardisation of the single-breath determination of carbon monoxide uptake in the lung. Eur Respir J 2005;26:720–735.

13. Viegi G, Baldi S, Begliomini E, Ferdeghini EM, Pistelli F. Single breath diffusing capacity for carbon monoxide: effects of adjustment for inspired volume dead space, carbon dioxide, hemoglobin and carboxy-hemoglobin. Respiration 1998;65:56–62.

14. Mohsenifar Z, Brown HV, Schnitzer B, Prause JA, Koerner SK. The effect of abnormal levels of hematocrit on the single breath diffusing capacity. Lung 1982;160:325–330.

15. Clark EH, Woods RL, Hughes JMB. Effect of blood transfusion on the carbon monoxide transfer factor of the lung in man. Clin Sci 1978;54:627–631.

16. Cotes JE, Dabbs JM, Elwood PC, Hall AM, McDonald A, Saunders MJ. Iron-deficiency anaemia: its effect on transfer factor for the lung (diffusing capacity) and ventilation and cardiac frequency during sub-maximal exercise. Clin Sci 1972;42:325–335.

17. Marrades RM, Diaz O, Roca J, et al. Adjustment of DLCO for hemo-globin concentration. Am J Respir Crit Care Med 1997;155:236–241.

18. Hancox B, Whyte K. Pocket Guide to Lung Function Tests, First Edition. McGraw-Hill, Sydney, 2001.

19. Pellegrino R, Viegi G, Enright P, et al. Interpretative strategies for lung function tests. Eur Respir J 2005;26:948–968.

20. Pride NB, Macklem PT. Lung mechanics in disease. In: Macklem PT, Mead J, eds. Handbook of Physiology. The Respiratory System. Mechanics of Breathing. Section 3, Vol. III, Part 2. American Physiological Society, Bethesda, MD, 1986;659–692.

21. Collard P, Njinou B, Nejadnik B, Keyeux A, Frans A. DLCO in stable asthma. Chest 1994;105:1426–1429.

22. Cotton DJ, Prabhu MB, Mink JT, Graham BL. Effects of ventilation inhomogeneity on DLCO SB-3EQ in normal subjects. J Appl Physiol 1992;73:2623–2630.

23. Cotton DJ, Prabhu MB, Mink JT, Graham BL. Effect of ventilation inhomogeneity on "intrabreath" measurements of diffusing capacity in normal subjects. J Appl Physiol 1993;75:927–932.

24. Gelb AF, Gold WM, Wright RR, Bruch HR, Nadel JA. Physiologic diagnosis of subclinical emphysema. Am Rev Respir Dis 1973;107:50–63.

25. Morrison NJ, Abboud RT, Ramadan F, et al. Comparison of single breath carbon monoxide diffusing capacity and pressure–volume curves in detecting emphysema. Am Rev Respir Dis 1989;139:1179–1187.

26. Bates DV. Uptake of CO in health and emphysema. Clin Sci 1952;11:21–32.

27. Hyatt RE, Scanlon PD, Nakamura M. Interpretation of Pulmonary Function Tests, A Practical Guide, Second Edition. Lippincott Williams & Wilkins, Philadelphia, PA, 2003.

28. Green M, Road J, Sieck GC, Similowski T. ATS/ERS statement on respiratory muscle testing: tests of respiratory muscle strength. Am J Respir Crit Care Med 2002;166:518–624.

29. Green M. Respiratory muscle testing. Bull Eur Physiol Respir 1984;20:433–436.
30. Salzman S. Pulmonary function testing. Tips on how to interpret the results. J Respir Dis 1999;20:809–822.
31. Gilbert R, Auchincloss JH. What is a "restrictive" defect? Arch Intern Med 1986;146:1779–1781.

Chapter 7
Illustrative Cases on PFT

Table 7.1 lists the normal values for the most important PFTs and their grading of severity.

CASE I

A 52-year-old female, Caucasian. Heavy smoker. History of chronic dyspnea.

1. Spirometry (Figure 7.1)

	Pred.	Pre	% Pred.	Post	% Change
FVC	3.34	1.53	46	2.31	50
FEV_1	2.70	0.41	15	0.53	30
FEV_1/FVC		0.27		0.23	
FEF_{25-75}	2.82	0.11	4	0.17	

2. Lung volumes

	Pred.	Pre	% Pred.
TLC	5.14	7.15	139
RV	1.86	5.20	280
RV/TLC	36%	73%	

3. Diffusing capacity

	Pred.	Pre	% Pred.
DL_{CO}	22.9	3.4	15
DL_{CO}/V_A	4.52	1.47	32
V_A	5.23	2.31	44

A. Altalag et al., *Pulmonary Function Tests in Clinical Practice*,
DOI: 10.1007/978-1-84882-231-3_7, © Springer-Verlag London Limited 2009

TABLE 7.1. PFT normal values and grading of severity scale*

Normal values (ATS) – apply mainly to young and middle ages

FVC	80–120 (% pred.)
FEV_1	80–120
FEV_1/FVC ratio	80–120
FEF_{25-75}	>65% pred. but can be as low as 55%
FEF_{25-75}/FVC ratio	>0.66 (more accurate)
TLC	80–120
FRC	75–120
RV	75–120
DL_{CO}	80–120
MEP	>90 cmH$_2$O
MIP	<–70 cmH$_2$O
Supine FVC	Within 10% of the sitting value; >30% drop suggests diaphragmatic paralysis

Traditional method for grading the severity of obstructive and restrictive disorders

Obstructive disorder (based on FEV_1) – ratio <0.7

May be a physiologic variant	FEV_1 100 (% pred.)
Mild	70–100
Moderate	60–69
Moderately severe	50–59
Severe	35–49
Very severe	<35

Restrictive disorder (based on TLC, preferred)

Mild	TLC >70 (% pred.)
Moderate	60–69
Severe	<60

Restrictive disorder (based on FVC, in case no lung volume study is available)

Mild	FVC >70 (% pred.)
Moderate	60–69
Moderately severe	50–59
Severe	35–49
Very severe	<35

*LLN can be applied to appropriate reference equations to determine an abnormal result

Technician's comments: Data acceptable and reproducible. Four puffs of salbutamol inhaler given.

Q1: Interpret this PFT.
Q2: What is the most likely diagnosis?
Q3: How can you estimate the volume of trapped air?

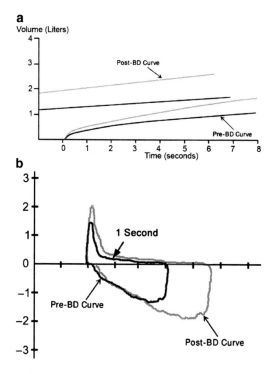

FIGURE 7.1. (**a**) VT curve; (**b**) FV curve.

INTERPRETATION

- Spirometry is obstructive:
  - VT curve:
    (a) Is flattened, suggesting obstructive defect. Notice that the FET (16 s) is prolonged, which supports the obstructive nature of the disorder.
    (b) The postbronchodilator curve shows a better morphology indicating a degree of bronchodilator response that needs to be defined numerically.
  - FV loop:
    (a) Is of a reasonable quality, although patient did not take full inspiration while measuring the IVC.
    (b) It is small and scooped out, with a "dog-leg appearance" (suggesting emphysema).

(c) The 1st second mark is closer to the leftmost end of the curve indicating a very low FEV_1 and FEV_1/FVC ratio, suggesting severe obstruction.

(d) Post-BD curve is bigger and less scalloped (suggesting some response to BD).

- Spirometric data:
  (a) Severe obstructive disorder ($\downarrow$ FEV_1 of a very severe range and very $\downarrow$ FEV_1/FVC ratio).
  (b) $\downarrow$ FEF_{25-75} supporting obstruction.
  (c) Partial but significant response to BD in FVC (780 ml and 50%). It did not reach significance in FEV_1 (120 ml and 30%).

Based on spirometry alone, the patient has a very severe obstructive defect with a significant response to bronchodilators. Given his smoking history and the dog-leg appearance in the FV curve, emphysema is the most likely but bronchial asthma cannot be excluded, which is supported by the significant response to BDs.

- Lung volume study is obstructive:
  - TLC and RV are $\uparrow$ with a very $\uparrow$ RV/TLC ratio suggesting emphysema with hyperinflation and air-trapping (in asthma TLC is usually normal).

Based on spirometry and lung volumes, both support obstruction, but emphysema is the most likely, as in asthma TLC is usually normal. DL_{CO} will be of help.

- DL_{CO}
  - DL_{CO}/V_A is extremely low suggesting a gas-exchange abnormality, favoring emphysema.
- Conclusion: very severe obstructive disorder with significant reversibility and impaired gas exchange suggesting emphysema.
  - Air-trapping can be estimated by two ways:
    (a) $TLC - V_A = 4.84$ L
    (b) RV (pred.) – RV (measured) = 3.34 L
  - This patient has severe emphysema clinically and radiologically.

CASE 2

A 74-year-old female, Caucasian.

1. Spirometry (Figure 7.2)

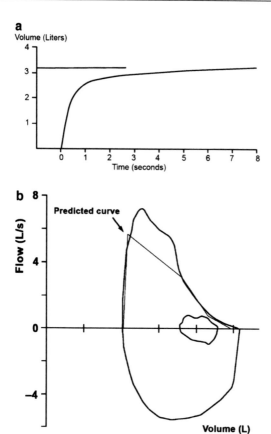

FIGURE 7.2. (a) VT curve; (b) FV curve.

	Pred.	Pre	% Pred.
FVC	3.21	3.17	99
FEV$_1$	2.38	2.57	108
FEV$_1$/FVC		81	
FEF$_{25-75}$	1.91	2.65	139

Technician's comments: Data acceptable and reproducible

Q1: Interpret this spirometry.

Q2: How would you describe the FV curve?

Interpretation

- Spirometry is normal:
  - VT curve looks normal. FET is ~12 s.
  - FV loop:
    (a) Is normal, with a knee. This is reproducible and considered a normal variant. Notice that PEF is normal.
  - Spirometric data:
    (a) Normal FEV_1, FVC, and ratio.
    (b) Normal FEF_{25-75}.
- Conclusion: normal study (the knee variant).

CASE 3

A 65-year-old female, Caucasian. History of progressive dyspnea.

1. Spirometry (Figure 7.3)

	Pred.	Pre	% Pred.
FVC	4.56	2.43	53
FEV_1	3.55	1.91	54
FEV_1/FVC		0.79	
FEF_{25-75}	3.27	1.55	47

Technician's comments: Data acceptable and reproducible.
Q1: Interpret this spirometry.
Q2: What is the most likely diagnosis?

Interpretation

- Spirometry is restrictive:
  - VT curve looks normal morphologically. There is no predicted curve to compare with.
  - FV loop:
    (a) Is small with a steep slope (witch's hat appearance). Its width (FVC) is clearly reduced with a preserved ratio.
    (b) PEF is preserved suggesting a parenchymal restriction.
    (c) The tidal FV loop is closer to the TLC, suggesting a true restriction (IC:ERV ratio is clearly <2:1).
  - Spirometric data:
    (a) Moderate restrictive disorder (Moderately reduced FVC with a normal ratio); ↓ FEF_{25-75} can be seen in restriction.
- Conclusion: spirometry is suggestive of a moderately severe restriction most likely due to an interstitial lung disease. A lung

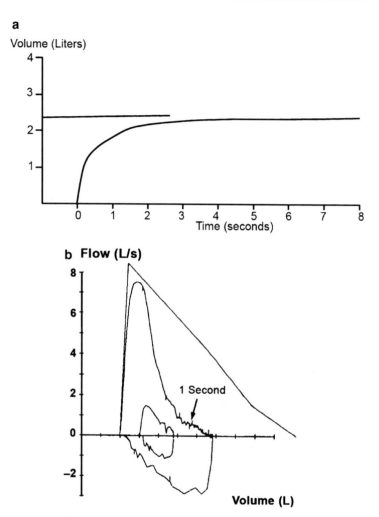

FIGURE 7.3. (**a**) VT curve; (**b**) FV curve.

volume study is indicated to confirm the restrictive nature of the disease (low TLC).
• This patient has lung fibrosis secondary to IPF.

CASE 4

A 79-year-old male, Asian. History of dyspnea.

1. Spirometry (Figure 7.4)

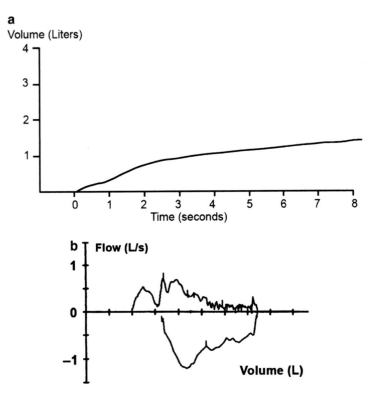

FIGURE 7.4. (**a**) VT curve; (**b**) FV curve.

	Pred.	Pre	% Pred.
FVC	3.02	1.37	45
FEV$_1$	2.34	0.61	26
FEV$_1$/FVC		48	
FEF$_{25-75}$	1.65	0.23	14

Technician's comments: Data acceptable and reproducible.
Q1: Interpret this spirometry.

Interpretation

- VT curve is very flat suggesting an obstructive disorder.
- FV loop is small and flat. It has flat inspiratory and expiratory components suggesting a fixed upper airway obstruction.
- This patient has a fibrotic tracheal stricture related to a previous tracheostomy.

CASE 5

A 54-year-old male, Caucasian.

1. Spirometry (Figure 7.5)

	Pred.	Pre	% Pred.	Post	% Change
FVC	5.11	4.70	90	4.61	-2
FEV$_1$	4.03	3.64	89	3.58	-1
FEV$_1$/FVC		78		77	
FEF$_{25-75}$	1.92	0.94	49		

2. Lung volumes

	Pred.	Pre	% Pred.
TLC	7.31	7.63	104
RV	2.21	2.58	117
RV/TLC	31	34	110
ERV	1.58	0.78	50

3. Diffusing capacity

	Pred.	Pre	% Pred.
DL$_{CO}$	30.50	27.99	92
DL$_{CO}$/V_A	4.34	4.19	96
V_A	7.02	6.68	95

Technician's comments: Data not reproducible. Best values reported. Four puffs of salbutamol inhaler given.

Q1: Interpret this PFT.

Q2: What is the most likely diagnosis?

Interpretation

- Spirometry is normal:
  - FV loop:
    (a) The pre-BD curve is interrupted by a cough in its 1st second. The study is not reproducible.
    (b) The curve looks normal and slightly smaller than the predicted one. FVC and the ratio look normal.
    (c) Post-BD curve is smaller than the pre-BD curve indicating lack of response to BDs.

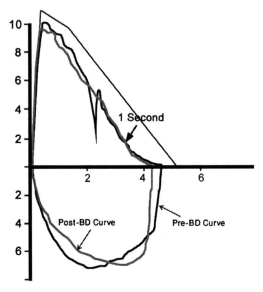

FIGURE 7.5. FV curve.

- Spirometric data:
  (a) FVC, FEV_1, and the ratio are normal with no response to BD.
  (b) ↓ FEF_{75} (non-specific and may be seen in obesity)

Based on spirometry alone, the patient has no significant obstructive or restrictive disorder despite the study quality.

- Lung volume study is normal except for an isolated reduction in ERV suggesting obesity.
- DL_{CO}
  - DL_{CO} and DL_{CO}/V_A are normal indicating that there is no gas-exchange abnormality.
- Conclusion: Normal PFT with isolated reduction in ERV suggestive of obesity. The patient's weight at the time of the test was 108 kg with a BMI of 33.

CASE 6
A 48-year-old female with chronic dyspnea. Spirometry (shown in Figure 7.6) was done in Body Box.

Technician's comments: Data acceptable and reproducible.

Q1: Interpret this FV curve

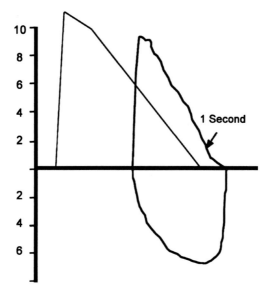

FIGURE 7.6. FV curve.

Interpretation

• FV loop morphology looks acceptable.
• It is small and has a steep slope (witch's hat).
• Its width (FVC) is low with normal ratio suggesting restriction.
• It is shifted to the right compared with the predicted indicating decreased TLC and RV, which is consistent with a restrictive defect secondary to an interstitial lung disease.
• This patient was found to have interstitial fibrosis secondary to sarcoidosis.

CASE 7
An 84-year-old male, Caucasian.

1. Spirometry (Figure 7.7)

	Pred.	Pre	% Pred.	Post	% Change
FVC	2.94	1.90	64	2.07	9
FEV$_1$	2.09	0.77	37	0.89	15
FEV$_1$/FVC		41		43	
FEF$_{25-75}$	1.44	0.22	15		

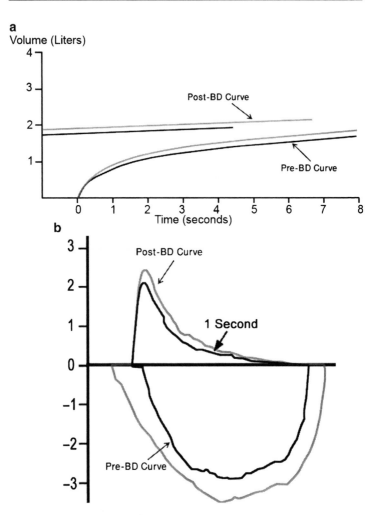

FIGURE 7.7. (**a**) VT curve; (**b**) FV curve.

Technician's comments: Data acceptable and reproducible. Four puffs of salbutamol inhaler given.
Q1: Interpret this spirometry.

Interpretation

• VT curve is flat with increased FET suggesting obstruction. The post-BD study indicates some improvement.

- FV loop:
  - Curve quality indicates either air leak or poor initial breath in the post-BD study.
  - Curve is small and scalloped indicating obstruction. The 1st second mark is very proximal indicating that FEV_1 and its ratio are very low.
  - Some improvement in the curve morphology following bronchodilators.
- Spirometric data:
  - FEV_1 and the ratio are severely decreased indicating a severe obstructive defect.
  - ↓ FEF_{75} is very low supporting obstruction
  - There is 15% improvement in FEV_1 but it is less than 200 ml (only 120 ml) indicating some response to BD that did not reach significance.
- Conclusion: Severe obstructive disorder with no response to BD.

CASE 8

A 61-year-old female, Caucasian. Unexplained SOB.

1. Spirometry

	Pred.	Pre	% Pred.	Post	% Change
FVC	2.85	2.47	87	2.55	3
FEV_1	2.27	2.13	94	2.17	2
FEV_1/FVC		86		85	
FEF_{25-75}	2.31	2.23	140	3.06	-5

2. Lung volumes

	Pred.	Pre	% Pred.
TLC	4.78	4.18	87
RV	1.92	1.71	89
RV/TLC	40	41	

3. Diffusing capacity

	Pred.	Pre	% Pred.
DL_{CO}	20.7	10.1	48.8
DL_{CO}/V_A	4.52	2.42	53.5
V_A	4.73	4.17	88

Technician's comments: Data acceptable and reproducible. Four puffs of salbutamol inhaler given.

Q1: Interpret this PFT.

Q2: What is the most likely diagnosis?

Interpretation

- Spirometry is normal with no response to bronchodilators.
- Lung volume study is normal.
- DL_{CO}/V_A is extremely low suggesting a gas-exchange abnormality.
- Conclusion: Isolated reduction in the diffusing capacity indicating an early parenchymal lung disease, pulmonary vascular disease, or anemia.
- This patient has pulmonary hypertension with a pulmonary artery systolic pressure of 74 mmHg.

CASE 9

A 61-year-old female, Caucasian.

1. Spirometry

	Pred.	Pre	% Pred.	Post	% Change
FVC	4.30	3.02	70	3.10	2
FEV_1	3.72	2.66	72	2.93	10
FEV_1/FVC		88		94	
FEF_{25-75}	4.41	2.65	60	3.46	31

2. Lung volumes

	Pred.	Pre	% Pred.
TLC	5.43	4.28	79
RV	1.15	1.50	130
RV/TLC	21%	35%	

3. Diffusing capacity

	Pred.	Pre	% Pred.
DL_{CO}	27.17	21.42	79
DL_{CO}/V_A	4.97	5.37	108
V_A	5.46	3.99	73

Technician's comments: Data acceptable and reproducible. Four puffs of salbutamol inhaler given.

Q1: Interpret this PFT.

Interpretation

- Spirometry is suggestive of mild restriction with some but insignificant response to bronchodilators.
- Lung volume study is obstructive but with a low TLC (making restriction alone less likely) and evidence of air trapping ($\uparrow$ RV).
- Diffusing capacity is normal.
- Conclusion: The spirometry is restrictive and the lung volume study is obstructive. The possibilities are either a combined defect (most likely) or an obstructive disorder with a suboptimal spirometry (unlikely as data are reproducible).
- This patient has emphysema and interstitial fibrosis.

CASE 10

A 55-year-old male, Caucasian, weight 84 kg; history of shortness of breath.

1. Spirometry (Figure 7.8)

	Pred.	Pre	% Pred.
FVC	4.73	5.00	106
FEV_1	3.75	3.25	87
FEV_1/FVC		79	
FEF_{25-75}	4.35	1.80	41
FIF_{50}		0.58	
FEF_{50}		2.42	

2. Lung volumes

	Pred.	Pre	% Pred.
TLC	6.91	6.73	97
RV	2.19	1.44	66
RV/TLC	0.31	0.21	68

3. Diffusing capacity

	Pred.	Pre	% Pred.
DL_{CO}	24.79	26.42	107
DL_{CO}/V_A	3.72	3.73	100

Technician's comments: Data acceptable and reproducible.
Q1: Interpret this PFT.

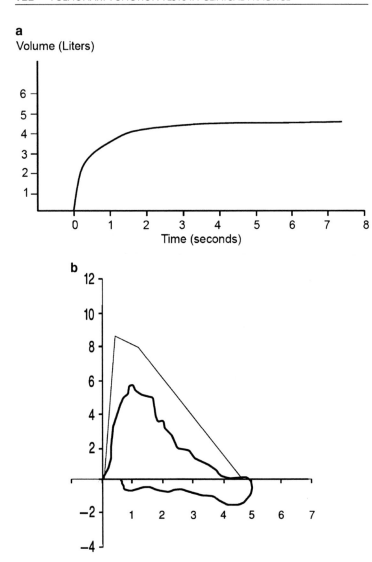

FIGURE 7.8. (a) VT curve; (b) FV curve.

Interpretation

- VT curve looks normal (no predicted curve to compare with).
- FV loop:
  - Curve quality looks suboptimal, which could be due to a disease state.

- Curve is small with a flat inspiratory component. This suggests a variable extrathoracic upper airway obstruction.
- The expiratory component of the curve is not significantly abnormal.
- Spirometric data:
  - Normal FVC, FEV_1, and FEV_1/FVC ratio.
  - $\downarrow FEF_{25-75}$ is non-specific.
  - FIF_{50}/FEF_{50} is much less than 1 indicating a variable extrathoracic upper airway obstruction.
- Lung volume study:
  - Normal TLC with low RV.
- DL_{CO} and DL_{CO}/V_A are normal.
- Conclusion: The only significant abnormality is the flattened inspiratory component of FV loop and a very low FIF_{50}/FEF_{50} ratio indicating a variable extrathoracic upper airway obstruction. This patient has laryngeal stenosis.

CASE 11

A 67-year-old male, Caucasian, weight 105 kg.

1. Spirometry (Figure 7.9)

	Pred.	Pre	% Pred.
FVC	4.36	2.66	61
FEV_1	3.38	2.05	61
FEV_1/FVC		77	
FEF_{25-75}	3.98	1.82	47

2. Lung volumes

	Pred.	Pre	% Pred.
TLC	6.79	4.82	71
RV	2.40	1.54	64
RV/TLC	0.35	0.32	92

3. Diffusing capacity

	Pred.	Pre	% Pred.
DL_{CO}	24.75	14.78	60
DL_{CO}/V_A	3.37	2.57	76

Technician's comments: Data acceptable and reproducible.
Q1: Interpret this PFT.

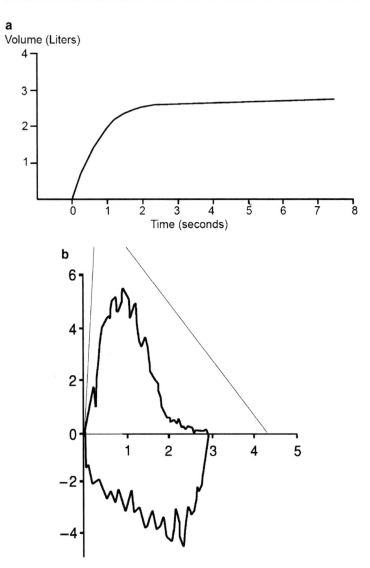

FIGURE 7.9. (a) VT curve; (b) FV curve.

Interpretation

- VT curve looks normal (no predicted curve to compare with).
- FV loop:

- Curve quality looks suboptimal with multiple variable efforts.
- The height (PEF) and width (FVC) of the curve are reduced.
- Spirometric data:
  - Reduced FVC and FEV_1 with a normal FEV_1/FVC ratio suggesting a possible restriction.
  - ↓ FEF_{25-75} is non-specific.
- Lung volume study:
  - Slightly reduced TLC with low RV confirming a mild restrictive pattern.
- DL_{CO} is low, which corrects partially when V_A is taken into consideration, which still cannot exclude a gas-exchange abnormality.
- Conclusion: Mild restrictive disorder. This patient has Parkinson's disease, which explains the variable effort noticed in the FV loop. The restrictive disorder noted is probably unrelated to Parkinson's disease.

CASE 12

A 64-year-old male, Caucasian, weight 120 kg; history of shortness of breath.

1. Spirometry

	Pred.	Pre	% Pred.
FVC	4.36	1.53	35
FEV_1	3.41	1.15	34
FEV_1/FVC		78	
FEF_{25-75}	3.95	0.87	22

2. Lung volumes

	Pred.	Pre	% Pred.
TLC	6.70	3.38	50
RV	2.40	1.54	64
RV/TLC	2.31	1.40	61

3. Diffusing capacity

	Pred.	Pre	% Pred.
DL_{CO}	26.73	16.04	60
DL_{CO}/V_A	4.23	4.72	112

Supine FVC: 0.97 L.
MIP: –27 cm water.
MEP: 229 cm water.

Technician's comments: Data acceptable and reproducible.
Q1: Interpret this PFT.

Interpretation

- Spirometric data:
  - Reduced FVC and FEV_1 with a normal FEV_1/FVC ratio suggesting a possible restriction.
  - ↓ FEF_{25-75} is non-specific.
- Lung volume study:
  - Significantly reduced TLC with a low RV confirming the restrictive nature of this disorder.
- DL_{CO} is low, which corrects when V_A is taken into consideration, which still cannot exclude a gas-exchange abnormality.
- Conclusion: Severe restrictive disorder with a relatively preserved DL_{CO} indicating a nonparenchymal cause of restriction.
- Further tests to be done include MEP and MIP, which showed a low MIP and normal MEP indicating inspiratory muscle (diaphragmatic) weakness. Supine FVC dropped significantly compared with the sitting value (>30% drop). This patient had a paralyzed diaphragm.

CASE 13
A 22-year-old male, Caucasian, weight 81 kg; history of shortness of breath.

1. Spirometry (Figure 7.10)

	Pred.	Pre	% Pred.
FVC	5.38	1.97	36
FEV_1	4.52	1.37	30
FEV_1/FVC		72	
FEF_{25-75}	4.99	1.14	23
PEF	9.24	1.68	18
FEF_{50}	5.73	1.51	26
FIF_{50}	5.38	1.80	33

2. Lung volumes

	Pred.	Pre	% Pred.
TLC	6.73	2.44	36
RV	1.47	0.23	16
RV/TLC	0.21	0.09	43

3. Diffusing capacity

	Pred.	Pre	% Pred.
DL_{CO}	36.67	20.34	55
DL_{CO}/V_A	5.46	7.82	143

Technician's comments: Data acceptable and reproducible.
Q1: Interpret this PFT.

Interpretation

- FV loop:
  - Is small and flat at both inspiratory and expiratory components, suggesting fixed upper airway obstruction.
- Spirometric data:
  - Reduced FVC and FEV_1 with a normal FEV_1/FVC ratio suggesting a restrictive disease.
  - Reduced PEF, FEF_{50}, and FIF_{50}. FIF_{50}/FEF_{50} ratio is around 1, which indicates a fixed upper airway obstruction.

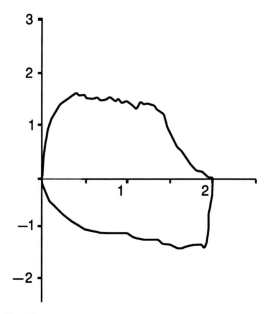

FIGURE 7.10. FV curve.

- Lung volume study:
  - Lung volumes are all significantly reduced confirming severe restriction.
- DL_{CO} is also low, which overcorrects when V_A is taken into consideration, which possibly indicates that there is no significant parenchymal abnormality.
- Conclusion: Fixed upper airway obstruction with severe restriction. This patient has lymphoma with significant paratracheal lymphadenopathy compressing the trachea. He was also found to have large bilateral pleural effusions related to his lymphoma causing this lung restriction.

CASE 14

A 54-year-old male, Caucasian, weight 89 kg; history of shortness of breath.

1. Spirometry (Figure 7.11)

	Pred.	Pre	% Pred.
FVC	4.27	2.74	64
FEV_1	3.45	1.98	58
FEV_1/FVC		72	
FEF_{25-75}	3.51	1.33	38
PEF	7.91	11.19	141

2. Lung volumes

	Pred.	Pre	% Pred.
TLC	6.28	4.07	65
RV	2.01	1.24	62
RV/TLC	32	30	

3. Diffusing capacity

	Pred.	Pre	% Pred.
DL_{CO}	28.19	18.26	65
DL_{CO}/V_A	6.28	3.97	63

Technician's comments: Data acceptable and reproducible.
Q1: Interpret this PFT.

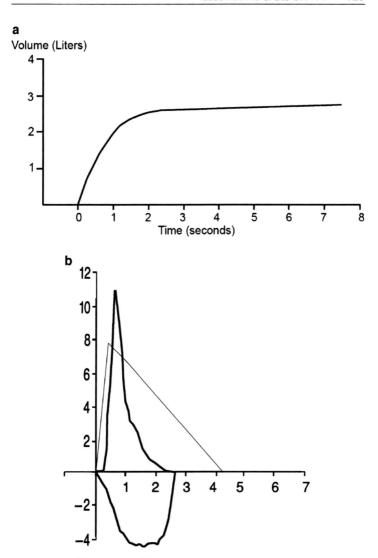

FIGURE 7.11. (**a**) VT curve; (**b**) FT curve.

Interpretation

- Spirometry is restrictive:
  - VT curve looks normal morphologically. There is no predicted curve to compare with.

- FV loop:
  - Is small with a steep slope (witch's hat appearance). Its width (FVC) is clearly reduced.
  - PEF is increased suggesting a parenchymal restriction.
- Spirometric data:
  - Reduced FVC and FEV_1 with a normal FEV_1/FVC ratio suggesting a restrictive disease.
- Lung volumes:
  - Moderately reduced TLC and RV with a preserved RV/TLC ratio confirming moderately severe restriction.
- DL_{CO}/V_A is reduced going with a parenchymal restriction.
- Conclusion: Moderately severe restrictive disorder most likely due to a parenchymal disease.

CASE 15

A 78-year-old male, Caucasian, weight 80 kg.

1. Spirometry (Figure 7.12)

	Pred.	Pre	% Pred.
FVC	4.06	2.46	61
FEV_1	3.07	1.33	43
FEV_1/FVC		54	
FEF_{25-75}	2.70	0.44	16
PEF	7.54	4.88	65

2. Lung volumes

	Pred.	Pre	% Pred.
TLC	6.67	5.00	75
RV	2.51	2.42	97
RV/TLC	38	48	127

3. Diffusing capacity

	Pred.	Pre	% Pred.
DL_{CO}	23.52	10.82	46
DL_{CO}/V_A	3.80	2.64	69

Technician's comments: Data acceptable and reproducible.

Q1: Interpret this PFT.

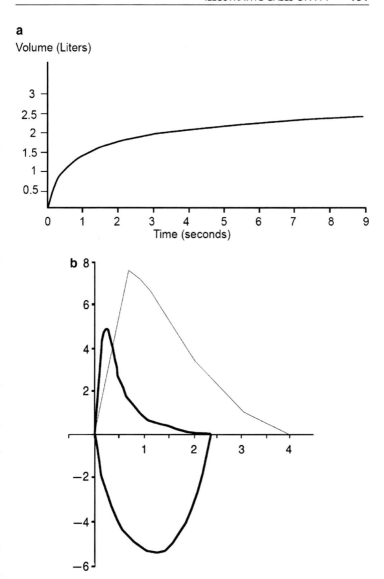

FIGURE 7.12.   (**a**) VT curve; (**b**) FV curve.

Interpretation

- Spirometry is obstructive:
  - VT curve looks flat. FET is 9 s.
  - FV loop:
    (a) The expiratory curve is small and scooped out, suggesting an obstructive disorder.
  - Spirometric data:
    (a) Reduced FVC and FEV_1 with a reduced FEV_1/FVC ratio suggesting a severe obstructive disorder. FEF_{25-75} is reduced going with an obstructive disorder.
- Lung volume study is restrictive:
  - Mildly reduced TLC with a normal RV and increased RV/TLC ratio. The reduced TLC indicates a restrictive disorder.
- DL_{CO}/V_A is reduced, which may be seen in both restrictive and obstructive disorders.
- Conclusion: Severe obstructive disorder with a mild restriction. This patient has emphysema and lung resection.

Chapter 8
Arterial Blood Gas Interpretation

INTRODUCTION

- If you are given this ABG with pH (7.38), $PaCO_2$ (41 mmHg), PaO_2 (95), HCO_3 (23 mmHg), Na^+ (143 mg/dl), and Cl^- (98 mg/dl), how would you interpret it?
- These values are all normal but the patient has significant acid–base disturbances that may be fatal, if untreated. This chapter tries to introduce a simple approach to help solving any acid–base problem including the hidden ones, such as the one given above.
- The above ABG is discussed in case number 4, later.

DEFINITIONS[1]

- *Acidosis* is a disturbance that lowers the extracellular fluid pH.
- *Alkalosis* is a disturbance that raises the extracellular fluid pH.
- *Acidemia* is a reduction of the final extracellular fluid pH. Accordingly an acidemia may result from a combination of different types of acidosis or a combination of acidosis and alkalosis.
- *Alkalemia* is an elevation of the final extracellular fluid pH.
- *Base excess (BE)* is the amount of acid (+) or base (–) (in mEq/L) required to restore the pH of a liter of blood to the normal range at a P_aCO_2 of 40 mmHg. Table 8.1 shows the normal values of the ABG components.

A. Altalag et al., *Pulmonary Function Tests in Clinical Practice*,
DOI: 10.1007/978-1-84882-231-3_8, © Springer-Verlag London Limited 2009

TABLE 8.1. ABG normal values

pH	7.35–7.45
P_aCO_2	35–45 mmHg
P_aO_2	>80 mmHg
HCO_3	21–26 mmol/L (Average: ~24)
BE	0 to –2 mmol/L
SaO_2	>95%
Anion gap (AG)	10 ± 4 (Average: ~12)
$P_{(A-a)}O_2$	<15

To convert from KPa (Kilo-Pascal) to mmHg, multiply by 7.5.

HENDERSON EQUATION[2]

- This equation represents the relationship between the components of the ABG and may be written in different ways*:
  - A simple way is as follows†:

$$[H^+] = K \times \frac{[H_2CO_3]}{[HCO_3]}, \text{ where } K = 24.$$

  - By substituting P_aCO_2 for $[H_2CO_3]$ that is measured from ABG, the equation can be written in a more practical way[2]:

$$[H^+] = K \times \frac{P_aCO_2}{[HCO_3]}, \text{ where } K = 24.$$

  - $[H^+]$ is the hydrogen ion (proton) concentration, and it can be easily calculated from pH; see Table 8.2.
  - The rest of the variables can be acquired directly from the ABG.
- The purpose of this equation is as follows:
  - To ensure that the ABG values are accurately recorded. Solving the equation should result in equalization of its two sides.

---

*Henderson equation is the equation shown earlier, while Henderson–Hasselbalch equation is a logarithmic expression of Henderson equation, shown here: pH = pK + log ($[HCO_3]/[H_2CO_3]$).[1]

†This equation is derived from the chemical reaction: $H_2CO_3 \leftrightarrow H^+ + HCO_3^-$, which can be written as: $[H^+] \leftrightarrow [H_2CO_3]/[HCO_3^-]$; therefore: $[H^+] = K \times [H_2CO_3]/[HCO_3^-]$, as K is the thermodynamic constant that varies with the temperature and ionic strength of the solution. In this case $K = 24$.

TABLE 8.2 Calculating [H+] from pH[2]

When pH is within (7.30–7.50)

pH of 7.40 $\leftrightarrow$ [H+] = 40 nmol/L

Then *increasing* or decreasing pH by 0.01 is equivalent to *decreasing* or increasing [H+] by 1 nmol/L, respectively (remember that [H+] changes in the opposite direction of pH; for instance, acidosis decreases pH but increases [H+]).

So if pH is 7.35, then [H+] will equal 40 + 5 = 45 nmol/L.

When pH is outside the range of 7.3–7.5, the following applies (Note, this technique can be applied when pH is within the above range too):

pH of 7.00 $\leftrightarrow$ [H+] = 100 nmol/L

Then every *increase* or decrease of pH by 0.10 is equivalent to *multiplying* or dividing [H+] by 0.8.

So if pH is 7.10, then [H+] will equal 100 × 0.8 = 80 nmol/L.

If pH is 7.20, then [H+] will equal 100 × 0.8 × 0.8 = 64 nmol/L.

If pH is 7.40, then [H+] = 100 × 0.8^4 = 40.

If pH is 6.80, then [H+] = 100/(0.8 × 0.8) = 156.

If you do not want to bother yourself with these boring calculations, the following table can be of help:

pH	[H+]	pH	[H+]
7.00	100	7.35	45
7.05	89	7.40	40
7.10	79	7.45	35
7.15	71	7.50	32
7.20	63	7.55	28
7.25	56	7.60	25
7.30	50	7.65	22

- If one of the ABG values is missing, the equation can be solved to determine that missing value. Indeed this is usually done for ABG results. The pH and P_aCO_2 are actually measured in the blood sample and the HCO_3 is calculated using this equation, e.g., pH 7.3 ([H+] = 50), P_aCO_2 = 50 mmHg, and HCO_3 = unknown.
- By applying Henderson equation:

$$[H^+] = K \times (P_aCO_2 / [HCO_3]),$$

$$[50 = 24 \times (50 / [HCO_3]).$$

Therefore, $[HCO_3]$ = 24.

METABOLIC ACIDOSIS

Causes

Metabolic acidosis can be classified – depending on the nature of the acid causing the disturbance – into anion gap (AG) and nonanion gap (NAG) metabolic acidosis.[8,9] The NAG metabolic acidosis is also called *hyperchloremic metabolic acidosis*, because it is associated with high serum chloride. Table 8.3 summarizes these causes.

TABLE 8.3 Causes of metabolic acidosis

Anion gap metabolic acidosis
Uremia
Ketoacidosis
   Diabetes
   Alcohol-induced
   Starvation
Lactic acidosis
Toxin ingestion
   Salicylates
   Methanol
   Ethylene glycol
   Paraldehyde

Nonanion gap (hyperchloremic) metabolic acidosis
GI loss of HCO_3
   Diarrhea
   Ileostomy or colostomy
   Uretero-segmoid fistula
   Pancreatic fistula
Renal loss of HCO_3
   Renal tubular acidosis
      Proximal (type II)
      Distal (types I and IV)
   Carbonic anhydrase inhibitors/deficiency
   Hypoaldosteronism, aldosterone inhibitors
   Hyperkalemia
   Renal tubular disease
      Acute tubular necrosis (ATN)
      Chronic tubulointerstitial disease
Iatrogenic
   Ammonium chloride (NH_4Cl)
   Hydrochloric acid (HCl) therapy
   Hyperalimentation (with TPN lacking acetate buffer)
   Dilutional acidosis (caused by excessive isotonic saline infusion)

Approach to Metabolic Acidosis

- In both types of metabolic acidosis, the primary disturbance is a drop in bicarbonate. Because the respiratory system is fast in its compensation, there is a rapid drop in P_aCO_2, which should always accompany a pure metabolic acidosis (remember that P_aCO_2 changes in the same direction as HCO_3 in a pure metabolic disturbance).[‡] Remember that normal bicarbonate does not exclude a metabolic disturbance as metabolic acidosis may coexist with metabolic alkalosis.
- We suggest a protocol in interpreting ABG. Table 8.4 summarizes a useful one.
- The first step is to determine the type of disturbance (acidemia or alkalemia) by looking at the pH.
- Then determine the most likely primary disturbance. So, if a reduction in HCO_3 is the predominant abnormality in the setting of acidemia, then the primary disturbance is a metabolic acidosis.
- Determine the type of metabolic acidosis you are dealing with (AG or NAG) by calculating the AG[18]:

$$AG = Na^+ - (Cl^- + HCO_3^-).$$

  – If normal (≤12), then this is a nonanion gap metabolic acidosis (NAGMA). Go to the next step.
  – If high (>12), then this is an anion gap metabolic acidosis (AGMA). In AGMA, you need to determine then whether

TABLE 8.4. Approach to ABG interpretation

Determine whether the ABG data are accurate by quickly applying Henderson equation.

Look at the pH and determine whether it is normal, acidemic, or alkalemic.

Determine the most likely primary disturbance (by looking at HCO_3 and P_aCO_2 and determining which one is largely responsible).

  If the primary disturbance is respiratory, determine whether it is acute or chronic.

  If the primary disturbance is metabolic, determine whether an appropriate respiratory compensation is present.

Calculate the AG.

Calculate the corrected HCO_3, if applicable.

[‡]P_aCO_2 in fact follows the pH (same direction as change in pH). Therefore, if P_aCO_2 fails to decrease (or if increased) in response to a decreased pH (e.g., secondary to metabolic acidosis), then a primary respiratory acidosis is diagnosed straight away.

another metabolic disturbance is present, by calculating the corrected HCO_3:

Corrected $HCO_3 = \Delta G +$ measured HCO_3 as $\Delta G = AG - 12$.

(a) If the corrected HCO_3 is *within* the normal range of HCO_3 (21–26), then there is no other metabolic disturbance, so go to the next step.

(b) If the corrected HCO_3 is *higher* than the normal range, then there is an additional metabolic alkalosis (corrected HCO_3 is higher than it should be).

(c) If the corrected HCO_3 is *lower* than the range, then there is an additional NAG metabolic acidosis (NAGMA).

• Determine whether there is a primary respiratory disturbance by initially looking at the P_aCO_2.

– If P_aCO_2 is normal or high (opposite direction to HCO_3), then there is a primary respiratory acidosis. Go to the next step.[§]

– If P_aCO_2 is low (same direction as HCO_3), then calculate the expected P_aCO_2 range[¶,10,11]:

Expected P_aCO_2 range $= 1.5$ x $HCO_3 + (8\pm2)$.

(a) If the patient's P_aCO_2 is *within* this range, then the patient has no respiratory disturbance (this is an appropriate compensation).

(b) If the patient's P_aCO_2 is *above* the range, then there is a primary respiratory acidosis (inadequate compensation).

(c) If the patient's P_aCO_2 is *below* the range, then there is a primary respiratory alkalosis (overcompensation). The lowest level P_aCO_2 can reach as a compensation for metabolic acidosis is 10–12 mmHg.[15]

• In NAGMA, determine whether the cause is of renal or nonrenal origin by calculating the urine anion gap (also called urine net charge or UNC)[21]:

Urine gap $= (U_{Na} + U_k) - U_{Cl}$.

– If the urine gap is *negative*, then the kidney is appropriately compensating by secreting H^+ in the form of ammonia

---

[§]If in doubt, calculate the expected P_aCO_2 range shown in the next point.

[¶]This formula is sometimes called Winters' equation.[11] Other methods to determine the expected P_aCO_2 include: (1) $P_aCO_2 = HCO_3 + 15$,[15] (2) P_aCO_2 should approximate the last two digits of pH in a steady state metabolic acidosis,[19] (3) or P_aCO_2 drops by ~1 mmHg for each 1 mEq/L drop in HCO_3.

TABLE 8.5. Approach to metabolic acidosis

Quickly apply the Henderson equation.

Look at the pH (normal, acidemia, or alkalemia).

The reduction in HCO_3 is the predominant abnormality → primary metabolic acidosis.

Calculate the AG (AG = Na^+ − (Cl^- + HCO_3))

If normal (~12) → nonanion gap metabolic acidosis (NAGMA).

If high (>12) → anion gap metabolic acidosis (AGMA). Calculate the corrected HCO_3 (Corrected HCO_3 = ΔG + measured HCO_3 as ΔG = AG − 12):

  − If within normal range of HCO_3 (21–26) → no other metabolic disturbance.

  − If >26 → primary metabolic alkalosis.

  − If <21 → primary nonanion gap metabolic acidosis.

Look at P_aCO_2:

If normal or high → primary respiratory acidosis. If in doubt, calculate expected P_aCO_2 range.

If low → calculate the expected P_aCO_2 range, given by 1.5 × HCO_3 + (8 ± 2):

  − If the patient's P_aCO_2 is within this range → no respiratory disturbance.

  − If patient's P_aCO_2 is above the range → primary respiratory acidosis.

  − If patient's P_aCO_2 is below the range → primary respiratory alkalosis.

In NAGMA, calculate urine anion gap (urine gap = (U_{Na} + U_K) − U_{Cl}):

If negative → extrarenal cause of metabolic acidosis.

If positive → a renal cause of the metabolic acidosis (RTA).

(NH_4^+), which neutralizes this negative urine anion gap. An extrarenal cause of metabolic acidosis is the most likely.

  − If the urine gap is *positive (or zero)*, then the kidneys are not secreting H^+ appropriately, indicating a renal cause of the metabolic acidosis [renal tubular acidosis (RTA)].

• These steps are summarized in Table 8.5.

METABOLIC ALKALOSIS

Causes

• Are classified into *Cl⁻-responsive* and *Cl⁻-resistant alkaloses*, which are summarized in Table 8.6.

Approach to Metabolic Alkalosis

• Similar to metabolic acidosis, metabolic alkalosis presents as a high HCO_3, which is compensated for by an increase in

TABLE 8.6. Causes of metabolic alkalosis

Cl responsive:
GI loss of H$^+$
    Vomiting, nasogastric suctioning
    Cl$^-$-rich diarrhea
    Villous adenoma
Renal loss of H$^+$
    Diuretics
    Hypovolemia
Posthypercapnia
High-dose carbenicillin

Cl resistant:
Renal loss of H$^+$
    Primary hyperaldosteronism
    Increased corticosteroid activity
        Primary hypercortisolism
        Adrenocorticotropic hormone (ACTH) excess
        Drug-induced
        Licorice ingestion
    Hypokalemia
    Increased renin activity (e.g., renin-secreting tumor)
Iatrogenic
    Excessive NaHCO$_3$ infusion
    Excessive citrate infusion (massive blood transfusion)
    Excessive acetate infusion (hyperalimentation with
        acetate-containing TPN)
    Excessive lactate infusion (Ringer's lactate)
    Milk–alkali syndrome

P_aCO_2[16,17] (which rarely exceeds a level of 60 mmHg[15]). A normal or a low P_aCO_2 indicates a respiratory alkalosis, in this setting.

- Determine the type of disturbance (acidemia or alkalemia) by looking at the pH.
- Then determine the most likely primary disturbance. So if the increase in HCO$_3$ is the predominant abnormality rather than a decrease in P_aCO_2, then the primary disturbance is metabolic alkalosis.
- Determine whether a primary metabolic acidosis is present as well by calculating AG:
  - If *normal* (~12), then there is no primary metabolic acidosis. Go to the next step.
  - If *high* (>12), then there is an additional primary AGMA.
- Determine whether there is a primary respiratory disturbance by initially looking at the P_aCO_2.

- If P_aCO_2 is *normal* or low (opposite direction to HCO_3), then there is a primary respiratory alkalosis. Go to next step.[||]
- If P_aCO_2 is *high* (same direction as HCO_3), then calculate the expected P_aCO_2 range[12–14]:

Expected P_aCO_2 range = 0.9 x HCO_3 + (9 to 16).

(a) If the patient's P_aCO_2 is *within* this range, then the patient has no additional respiratory disturbance (this is an appropriate compensation).
(b) If the patient's P_aCO_2 is *above* the range, then there is a primary respiratory acidosis (overcompensation).
(c) If the patient's P_aCO_2 is *below* the range, then there is a primary respiratory alkalosis (inadequate compensation).
- Determine the type of metabolic alkalosis (Cl^- responsive or Cl^- resistant) by measuring the urinary Cl^- (U_{Cl})[1]:
  - If U_{Cl} is <20 mmol/l, then this is Cl^- responsive (depleted) metabolic alkalosis. Think of it as the body is trying to conserve Cl^-.
  - If U_{Cl} is >20 mmol/l, then this is Cl^- resistant (expanded) metabolic alkalosis.
- Table 8.7 summarizes these steps.

TABLE 8.7. Approach to metabolic alkalosis

Quickly apply the Henderson equation.
Look at the pH (normal, acidemia, or alkalemia).
The increase in HCO_3 is the predominant abnormality → primary metabolic alkalosis.
Calculate the AG (AG = Na^+– (Cl^- + HCO_3)):
    If normal (~12) → no primary metabolic acidosis.
    If high (>12) → primary anion gap metabolic acidosis (AGMA).
Look at P_aCO_2:
    If normal or low → primary respiratory alkalosis. If in doubt, calculate
        expected P_aCO_2 range.
    If high → calculate the expected P_aCO_2 range, which is equal to 0.9 ×
HCO_3 + (9 to 16):
        – If patient's P_aCO_2 is within this range → no respiratory disturbance.
        – If patient's P_aCO_2 is above the range → primary respiratory acidosis.
        – If patient's P_aCO_2 is below the range → primary respiratory alkalosis.
Check the urinary Cl^- (U_{Cl}):
    If <20 mmol/l → Cl^- responsive metabolic alkalosis.
    If >20 mmol/l → Cl^- resistant metabolic alkalosis.

[||]If in doubt, calculate the expected P_aCO_2 range shown in the next point.

RESPIRATORY ACIDOSIS

Types of Respiratory Acidosis

- Because the body compensates slowly for a primary respiratory disturbance, the latter is then classified into acute and chronic forms. The following will highlight these forms.
- In acute respiratory acidosis, for every 10 mmHg rise in P_aCO_2[3]:
  - pH drops by 0.08, that is:

$$\text{pH} = 0.08 \times \frac{P_aCO_2 - 40}{10}$$

  - HCO_3 increases by 1 mmol/L; maximum level of HCO_3 is ~32 mmHg.
- In chronic respiratory acidosis, for every 10 mmHg rise in P_aCO_2[4]:
  - pH drops by 0.03, that is:

$$\text{pH} = 0.03 \times \frac{P_aCO_2 - 40}{10}.$$

  - HCO_3 increases by 3 mmol/L; maximum level of HCO_3 is ~45 mmHg.
- Tables 8.8 and 8.9 summarize the causes and steps of interpretation of respiratory acidosis, respectively.

TABLE 8.8. Causes of respiratory acidosis

Obstructive Disorders
Upper airway obstruction
    Foreign body
    Laryngospasm
    Obstructed endotracheal tube
    Obstructive sleep apnea
Lower airway obstruction
    Severe bronchospasm due to bronchial asthma or COPD

Restrictive disorders (see Table 1.7)
ILD
Chest wall restriction
Loss of air spaces (pleural effusion, pneumothorax)
Pleural disease

Hypoventilation
Central (e.g., secondary to sedative and narcotic drugs)

(continued)

TABLE 8.8. (continued)

Obesity-hypoventilation syndrome
Neuromuscular disease (Table 5.1)

Parenchymal lung disease (like ARDS)

Increased CO$_2$ production
Fever, shivering
Hypermetabolism
High carbohydrate diet

Others
Inappropriate ventilator settings
Compensatory

TABLE 8.9. Approach to respiratory acidosis

Quickly apply the Henderson equation.
Look at the pH (normal, acidemia, or alkalemia).
The increase in P_aCO_2 is the predominant abnormality → primary respiratory acidosis.
Determine whether acute or chronic

Acute: pH ↓ by 0.08 for every 10 mmHg ↑ in P_aCO_2; HCO$_3$ ↑ by 1 mmol/L (max ~32).
Chronic: pH ↓ by 0.03 for every 10 mmHg ↑ in P_aCO_2; HCO$_3$ ↑ by 3 mmol/L (max ~45).

Calculate the AG (AG = Na$^+$ − (Cl$^-$ + HCO$_3$))
   If high (>12) → primary anion gap metabolic acidosis (AGMA).
      If applicable, calculate the Corrected HCO$_3$, as in metabolic acidosis.
   If normal (~12) → Look at HCO$_3$.
      If ↓ or N → primary nonanion gap metabolic acidosis.
      If ↑ → look at HCO$_3$ and determine the type of respiratory acidosis:
      (HCO$_3$ ↑ by 1 (acute) *or* 3 (chronic) for each 10 mmol/L ↑ in P_aCO_2)
      If within the expected → no primary metabolic disturbance.
      If lower → nonanion gap metabolic acidosis.
      If higher → metabolic alkalosis.

RESPIRATORY ALKALOSIS

Types of Respiratory Alkalosis

- In acute respiratory alkalosis, for every 10 mmHg drop in P_aCO_2[5]:
  - pH rises by 0.08, that is:

$$pH = 0.08 \times \frac{40 - P_aCO_2}{10}$$

TABLE 8.10. Causes of respiratory alkalosis

Increased hypoxemic drive
Right-to-left shunt
High altitude

Pulmonary disease
Emphysema
Pulmonary embolism
Pulmonary congestion

Stimulation of respiratory center
Anxiety, pain, psychogenic
Liver failure with encephalopathy
Fever, Sepsis, infection
Respiratory stimulants (e.g., salicylates, progesterone)
Pregnancy

Others
Inappropriate ventilator settings
Compensatory

TABLE 8.11. Approach to respiratory alkalosis

Quickly apply the Henderson equation.
Look at the pH (normal, acidemia, or alkalemia).
The drop in $P_a CO_2$ is the predominant abnormality → primary respiratory alkalosis.
Determine whether acute or chronic
    Acute: pH ↑ by 0.08 (and HCO_3 ↓ by 2 mmol/L) for every 10 mmHg ↓ in $P_a CO_2$.
    Chronic: pH ↑ by 0.03 (and HCO_3 ↓ by 5–7 mmol/L) for every 10 mmHg ↓ in $P_a CO_2$.
Calculate the AG (AG = Na^+ − (Cl^- + HCO_3))
    If high (>12) → primary anion gap metabolic acidosis (AGMA).
        If applicable, calculate the Corrected HCO_3, as in metabolic acidosis.
    If normal (~12) → Look at HCO_3.
        If ↑ or N → primary metabolic alkalosis.
        If ↓ → look at HCO_3 and determine the type of respiratory alkalosis
            (HCO_3 ↓ by 2 (acute) *or* 5–7 (chronic) for each 10 mmol/L ↓ in $P_a CO_2$).
            If within the expected → no primary metabolic disturbance.
            If lower → nonanion gap metabolic acidosis
            If higher → metabolic alkalosis.

   – HCO_3 drops by 2 mmol/L.
• In chronic respiratory alkalosis, for every 10 mmHg drop in $P_a CO_2$[6,7]:
   – pH drops by 0.03, that is:

$$pH = 0.03 \times \frac{40 - P_a CO_2}{10}$$

- HCO_3 increases by 5–7 mmol/L.
- Tables 8.10 and 8.11 summarize the causes and steps of interpretation of respiratory alkalosis, respectively.

EFFECT OF A LOW ALBUMIN LEVEL ON AG

- Because albumin is one of the unmeasured anions in the blood, a drop in its level (e.g., secondary to a critical illness or liver disease) will influence the AG level. In this case, the calculated AG should be adjusted for albumin**:

    Adjusted AG = Calculated AG + [2.5 × (4.5 − alb in g/dl)].

- If this adjustment is ignored with a low albumin, the calculated anion gap will be underestimated and a significant AGMA may be missed.

ACID–BASE NOMOGRAM

- The nomogram shown in Figure 8.1 is one of many acid–base nomograms developed to assist in solving difficult acid–base disturbances and involves plotting pH, HCO_3, and P_aCO_2.[20] These are commonly referred to as Flenley's acid–base nomograms.

THE ALVEOLAR–ARTERIAL (A–a) OXYGEN GRADIENT AND ALVEOLAR GAS EQUATION[23]

Alveolar Gas Equation[††]

- This equation allows us to estimate the O_2 tension in the alveoli (P_AO_2):

$$P_AO_2 = P_IO_2 - \frac{P_aCO_2}{RQ}, \text{where } P_IO_2 = F_IO_2(P_{atm} - P_{H_2O}).$$

** This equation can also be written as follows: Adjusted AG = Calculated AG + [0.25 × (45 − alb in g/L)].

†† Abbreviations: P_AO_2 is the O_2 tension in the alveoli; P_aO_2 is the O_2 tension in the arterial blood; P_IO_2 is the O_2 tension in the inspired air; $P_{atm}O_2$ is the O_2 tension in the atmospheric air; P_{H2O} is the partial pressure of water vapor; $P_{(A-a)}O_2$ is the alveolar–arterial O_2 gradient; P_ACO_2 is the CO_2 tension in the alveoli; P_aCO_2 is the CO_2 tension in the arterial blood; F_IO_2 is the fractional inspired O_2; RQ is the respiratory quotient.

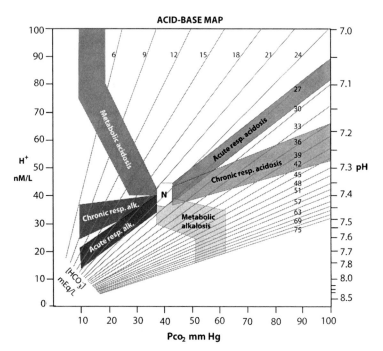

FIGURE 8.1. An acid–base nomogram, used to interpret ABG by directly plotting HCO₃, PaCO₂, and pH (With permission from Goldberg et al.[20])

- To understand this equation it is good to go through certain definitions:
  - $P_{atm}O_2$ is the atmospheric O_2 tension or partial pressure of O_2. It is calculated by multiplying the atmospheric pressure (760 mmHg at sea level) by the percentage of O_2 in the atmosphere (21%):

  $$P_{atm}O_2 = 0.21 \times P_{atm} = 0.21 \times 760 = 160 \text{mmHg(at sea level)}.$$

  - P_IO_2 is the O_2 tension of inspired air. Because the inspired air contains water vapor, it does not equal $P_{atm}O_2$. The water vapor tension (P_{H_2O}) should then be extracted from the atmospheric pressure before applying the earlier equation:

  $$P_IO_2 = F_IO_2 \times (P_{atm} - P_{H_2O}) = 0.21 \times (760 - 47) = 0.21 \times 713 = 150 \text{ mmHg}.$$

  (if breathing room air, at sea level)

- P_AO_2 is the alveolar O_2 tension. CO_2 diffuses from the circulation into the alveoli and hence reduces the P_AO_2. Accordingly, P_ACO_2 has to be subtracted from P_IO_2 to get P_AO_2. P_aCO_2 can be substituted for P_ACO_2 (when taking the respiratory quotient (RQ) into consideration, which is assumed to be 0.8 while at rest):

$$P_AO_2 = P_IO_2 - \frac{P_aCO_2}{RQ}, \text{ as RQ} = 0.8$$

$$= 150 - \frac{P_aCO_2}{0.8} \text{ OR } 150 - (P_aCO_2 \times 1.25),$$

$$= 150 - (40 \times 1.25) = 100 \text{ mm Hg.}$$

(if breathing room air, at sea level)

- P_aO_2 is the arterial O_2 tension that is measured in the ABG.
- F_IO_2 is the *fractional inspired O_2*, i.e., the percentage of O_2 in the inspired air. If breathing room air at sea level, it equals 0.21. This value changes if the patient is breathing through a nasal cannula or a face mask.
- *RQ* is the *respiratory quotient* and represents the amount of CO_2 produced for a given amount of O_2 consumed by our bodies. It equals 0.8 at rest, in a normal individual (because we produce 0.8 mole of CO_2 for each mole of O_2 we consume while at rest). The RQ increases with exercise, however. Next chapter discusses this in more detail.

A–a Gradient ($P_{(A-a)}O_2$)

- It is the difference between the alveolar and the arterial O_2 tension. Its calculation is now easy; see Figure 8.2:

$$P_{(A-a)}O_2 = P_AO_2 - P_aO_2, \text{ where } P_AO_2 = P_IO_2 - \frac{P_aCO_2}{RQ}$$

or

$$P_{(A-a)}O_2 = \left[P_IO_2 - \frac{P_aCO_2}{RQ} \right] - P_aO_2 \, .$$

- If at sea level and breathing room air (F_IO_2 of 0.21), then the equation can be simply written as follows:

$$P_{(A-a)}O_2 = \left[150 - \frac{P_aCO_2}{0.8} \right] - P_aO_2$$

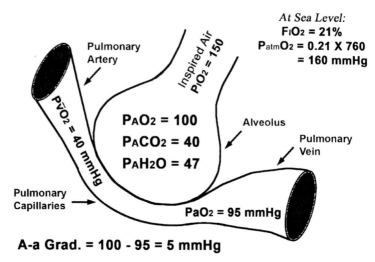

At Sea Level:
FiO2 = 21%
PatmO2 = 0.21 X 760
= 160 mmHg

Pulmonary
Artery

Inspired Air
PiO2 = 150

PvO2 = 40 mmHg

PAO2 = 100
PACO2 = 40
PAH2O = 47

Alveolus

Pulmonary
Vein

Pulmonary
Capillaries

PaO2 = 95 mmHg

A-a Grad. = 100 - 95 = 5 mmHg

FIGURE 8.2. This diagram summarizes the alveolar gas principles. Breathing RA at sea level in a normal person.

or

$$P_{(A-a)}O_2 = [150 - (1.25 \times P_aCO_2)] - P_aO_2$$

- $P_{(A-a)}O_2$ is normally ≤15 mmHg and increases with age. Different formulas are used to determine the normal $P_{(A-a)}O_2$ in relation to age; the following is a popular one[22]:

  Normal $P_{(A-a)}O_2$ = 2.5 + (0.21 × age in years).

MECHANISMS OF HYPOXEMIA[‡, 23]

These mechanisms can be classified into hypoxemia with a wide A–a gradient and hypoxemia with a normal A–a gradient:

- Hypoxemia with a wide A–a gradient ($P_{(A-a)}O_2 > 15$)
  - Shunting, like intracardiac shunts or pulmonary AV malformation
  - VQ mismatch, as in atelectasis
  - Decreased mixed venous O_2 tension ($P_{\bar{v}}O_2$)
  - Diffusion limitation (seen in severe ILD)

---

‡ Hypoxemia refers to a reduction in oxygen level in the blood while hypoxia refers to a reduction in oxygen at the tissue level.

- Hypoxemia with a normal A–a gradient ($P_{(A-a)}O_2 \leq 15$)
  - Low inspired O_2 ($\downarrow F_iO_2$), as in the case of high altitude.
  - Hypoventilation, as in obesity hypoventilation syndrome.
    (a) Hypoventilation causes primarily hypercapnia because of impaired washout of CO_2. As the alveolar CO_2 equals the arterial CO_2, both P_aCO_2 and P_ACO_2 will be equally elevated.
    (b) Hypoventilation causes hypoxemia, as well, if the patient is breathing room air. In this case, the degree of hypoxemia can be predicted from the level of P_aCO_2 using the alveolar gas equation. In general, if P_aCO_2 increases by 20 mmHg, P_AO_2 drops by 25 mmHg, even if the lungs are normal; Figure 8.3.[§§,#]

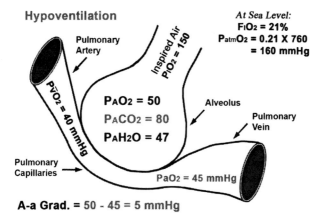

Hypoventilation

At Sea Level:
$FiO_2 = 21\%$
$P_{atm}O_2 = 0.21 \times 760$
$= 160$ mmHg

Pulmonary Artery

Inspired Air $P_iO_2 = 150$

$PVO_2 = 40$ mmHg

$PaO_2 = 50$
$PaCO_2 = 80$
$PaH_2O = 47$

Alveolus

Pulmonary Vein

Pulmonary Capillaries

$PaO_2 = 45$ mmHg

A-a Grad. = 50 - 45 = 5 mmHg

FIGURE 8.3. Effects of hypoventilation on alveolar and arterial O_2 and CO_2 tension: This patient is breathing room air at sea level and has a normal A–a gradient but still has a severe hypoxemia (P_aO_2 of 45). The reason for this hypoxemia is the elevated P_ACO_2 (secondary to hypoventilation). The P_ACO_2 has increased by 40 mmHg resulting in a reduction in P_AO_2 by 50 mmHg, which resulted in this degree of hypoxemia: $P_AO_2 = 150 - (1.25 \times 80) = 150 - 100 = 50$ mm Hg.

[§§] If P_aCO_2 is increased by 20 mmHg (i.e., P_aCO_2 of 60 mmHg), then P_AO_2 is calculated to be 75 mmHg using the alveolar gas equation (i.e., it dropped by 25 mmHg). So if P_aCO_2 is increased by 20 mmHg, P_AO_2 decreases by 25 mmHg; Figure 8.3. This rule is true only if the patient is breathing room air, at sea level.

[#] Another way of roughly predicting the degree of hypoxemia secondary to hypoventilation when the patient is breathing room air is the 130 rule. It simply states that the sum of P_aO_2 & P_aCO_2 should always equal 130 if the patient is breathing room air, at sea level. So, if P_aCO_2 is 80 mmHg then P_aO_2 should roughly be 130 – 80, i.e. 50 mmHg.

TYPES OF RESPIRATORY FAILURE 23

- *Type I respiratory failure* (hypoxemic respiratory failure) is characterized by hypoxemia and defined as an isolated reduction of P_aO_2 to <60 mmHg (the point at which the S_aO_2 drops steeply as shown in the O_2 dissociation curve); Figure 8.4. This type of respiratory failure is associated with an increased A–a gradient.
- *Type II respiratory failure* (ventilatory failure) is characterized by hypoxemia and hypercapnia and defined as a P_aCO_2 of >50 mmHg. The A–a gradient is normal.

ILLUSTRATIVE CASES
Case I

- A 63-year-old man presented with generalized malaise. His ABG showed pH (7.32), P_aCO_2 (24), HCO_3 (12), Na^+ (135), K^- (5.4), Cl^- (101). What type of acid–base disturbance this patient has?
- Interpretation:
  - Applying Henderson equation:

$$[H^+] = K(P_aCO_2 / [HCO_3]) \leftrightarrow 48 = 24(24 / 12) = 48.$$

  - So, the equation proves that the values are accurate.
  - pH is ↓, so this is an acidemia.

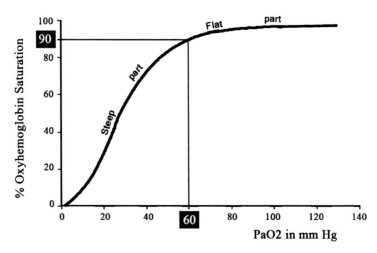

FIGURE 8.4. O_2 dissociation curve: when P_aO_2 > 60 mmHg, SaO_2 changes slightly with any given change in P_aO_2. When P_aO_2 < 60 mmHg, SaO_2 changes significantly with any given change in P_aO_2

- The predominant abnormality is the $\downarrow$ HCO_3 $\rightarrow$ so this is primary metabolic acidosis.
- By calculating the AG = Na^+ – (Cl^- + HCO_3) = 22 ($\uparrow$). It is >12 $\rightarrow$ so this is an AGMA.
- Corrected HCO_3 = ΔG + measured HCO_3 (as ΔG = AG – 12 = 10).
- So corrected HCO_3 = 10 + 12 = 22; it is within the normal range of HCO_3 (21–26), so there is no other metabolic disturbance.
- P_aCO_2 is low, so we should calculate the expected P_aCO_2 range:
- Expected P_aCO_2 range = 1.5 × HCO_3 + (8 ± 2)
- So, the expected P_aCO_2 range = 24–28; the patient's P_aCO_2 lies within this range, so there is no primary respiratory disturbance.
- Conclusion: This patient has a pure AGMA. This patient was found to have a creatinine of 500 mg/dl and so the unmeasured anions producing the gap were related to renal failure.

Case 2

- Interpret the following ABG: pH (7.11), P_aCO_2 (16), HCO_3 (5), Na^+ (133), Cl^- (118).
- Interpretation:
  - Applying Henderson equation indicates accurate results.
  - $\downarrow$ pH $\rightarrow$ so this is an acidemia.
  - $\downarrow$ HCO_3 $\rightarrow$ so this is a primary metabolic acidosis.
  - AG = Na^+ – (Cl^- + HCO_3) = 10 (normal) $\rightarrow$ so this is a NAGMA.
  - Expected P_aCO_2 range = 1.5 × HCO_3 + (8 ± 2) = 13.5–17.5 $\rightarrow$ the patient's P_aCO_2 lies within this range, so there is no primary respiratory disturbance.
  - Conclusion: The patient has a simple NAGMA. This patient is a 74-year-old very anxious lady who presented with severe gastroenteritis (diarrhea).

Case 3

- Interpret the following ABG: pH (6.88), P_aCO_2 (40), HCO_3 (7), Na^+ (135), Cl^- (118).
- Interpretation:
  - Applying Henderson equation indicates accurate results.
  - $\downarrow$ pH $\rightarrow$ so this is acidemia.
  - $\downarrow$ HCO_3 $\rightarrow$ so this is primary metabolic acidosis.
  - AG = Na^+ – (Cl^- + HCO_3) = 10 (normal) $\rightarrow$ so this is a NAGMA.

- P_aCO_2 is normal (it should be low in the face of a very low pH) → so, there is a *primary respiratory acidosis*. Although unnecessary you can still apply the equation – expected P_aCO_2 range = $1.5 \times HCO_3 + (8 \pm 2) = 16.5$–$20.5$ → the patient's P_aCO_2 is higher than this range so there is primary respiratory acidosis.
- Conclusion: A combined NAGMA and respiratory acidosis. This is the same patient described in case 2 after she was sedated with a benzodiazepine that suppressed her respiratory center. Sedation can be harmful in elderly patients.

Case 4

- A 23-year-old man presented with generalized malaise and vomiting. His ABG showed pH (7.38), P_aCO_2 (41), P_aO_2 (95), HCO_3 (23), Na^+ (143), Cl^- (98). What type of acid–base disturbance this patient has?
- Interpretation:
  - Applying Henderson equation indicates accurate results.
  - Normal pH → so no acidemia or alkalemia.
  - Normal HCO_3 → so no obvious metabolic abnormality.
  - AG = $Na^+ - (Cl^- + HCO_3) = 22$ (↑) → so there is an AGMA.
  - Corrected $HCO_3 = \Delta G$ + measured HCO_3 ($\Delta G = 22 - 12 = 10$).
  - So, the corrected $HCO_3 = 10+23 = 33$ → it is higher than the normal range of HCO_3 (21–26) → so there is an additional *metabolic alkalosis*.
  - P_aCO_2 is normal (so does the pH and HCO_3, so this is appropriate. If in doubt, apply expected P_aCO_2 range).
  - Expected P_aCO_2 range = $1.5 \times HCO_3 + (8 \pm 2) = 41$–$45$ → the patient's P_aCO_2 (41) lies within this range → so, there is no primary respiratory disturbance.
  - Conclusion: Although this ABG looked normal, a combined disturbance is present – AGMA and metabolic alkalosis. This patient was found to have a blood sugar of 510 mg/dl and ketones in the urine. He had diabetic ketoacidosis responsible for his AGMA and vomiting caused his metabolic alkalosis.

Case 5

- Interpret this ABG: pH (7.55), P_aCO_2 (49), HCO_3 (42), Na^+ (148), Cl^- (84).
- Interpretation:
  - Applying Henderson equation indicates accurate results.

- $\uparrow$ pH $\rightarrow$ so there is an alkalemia.
- $\uparrow$ HCO_3 $\rightarrow$ so there is a *metabolic alkalosis*.
- AG = Na^+ – $(Cl^-$ + $HCO_3)$ = 22 ($\uparrow$) $\rightarrow$ so there is an AGMA.
- $\uparrow$ P_aCO_2 (same direction as HCO_3) $\rightarrow$ Expected P_aCO_2 range = 0.9 × HCO_3 + (9 to 16) = 47–54 $\rightarrow$ the patient's P_aCO_2 (49) lies within this range $\rightarrow$ so, there is no primary respiratory disturbance.
- Conclusion: A combined AGMA and metabolic alkalosis with an alkalemic pH.

Case 6

- A 58-year-old man (heavy smoker) admitted to the ICU with sepsis. He is not intubated yet but has an NG tube. His ABG showed pH (6.88), P_aCO_2 (40), HCO_3 (7), Na^+ (142), Cl^- (100). What type of acid–base disturbance does this patient have?
- Interpretation:
  - Applying the Henderson equation indicates accurate results.
  - $\downarrow$ pH $\rightarrow$ so this is an acidemia.
  - $\downarrow$ HCO_3 $\rightarrow$ so this is a *primary metabolic acidosis*.
  - AG = Na^+ – $(Cl^-$ + $HCO_3)$ = 35 ($\uparrow$) $\rightarrow$ so this is an AGMA.
  - Corrected HCO_3 = 30; it is higher than the normal range of HCO_3 (21–26), so there is an additional *primary metabolic alkalosis*.
  - P_aCO_2 is normal (it should be low) $\rightarrow$ there is a *primary respiratory acidosis*.
  - Conclusion: A combined AGMA, metabolic alkalosis, and respiratory acidosis. This patient's metabolic acidosis is most likely related to sepsis. His respiratory acidosis is likely due to respiratory failure (COPD ± aspiration) and the metabolic alkalosis is due to gastric suction.

Case 7

- Interpret the following ABG: pH (7.55), P_aCO_2 (44), HCO_3 (45), Na^+ (144), Cl^- (112).
- Interpretation:
  - Applying Henderson equation:

$$[H^+] = K \times (P_aCO_2 / [HCO_3]) \leftrightarrow 28 \neq 24 \times (44 / 45) = 21.$$

So, the equation indicates that the values are incorrect. Repeat ABG sampling is advised or check with the lab to ensure accurate calculation of HCO_3 and recording of results.

Case 8

- A 68-year-old man known to have COPD presented to the emergency department with increasing cough. His ABG showed pH (7.34), P_aCO_2 (60), P_aO_2 (60), HCO_3 (31), AG (11). What is the acid–base disturbance? What is the A–a gradient provided that the patient was on room air, at sea level?
- Interpretation:
  - Applying Henderson equation indicates accurate results.
  - pH is slightly low indicating a mild acidemia.
  - ↑ P_aCO_2 → so this is a *primary respiratory acidosis*.
  - Metabolic compensation indicates a chronic respiratory acidosis: P_aCO_2 increased by 20 mmHg, which corresponds to a drop in pH by ~0.6 (0.3/10 mmHg of P_aCO_2) and an increase in HCO_3 by ~6 (3/10 mmHg of P_aCO_2).
  - AG is normal and HCO_3 is adequately increased → no metabolic disturbances.
  - The A–a gradient = $(150 - P_aCO_2 \times 1.25) - P_aO_2 = 15$ (normal)
  - Conclusion: Chronic primary respiratory acidosis.

Case 9

- The patient in case 8 became drowsy and unresponsive 4 h after presentation. A repeated ABG showed pH (7.15), P_aCO_2 (96), P_aO_2 (169), HCO_3 (33), AG (10).
- Interpretation:
  - Applying Henderson equation indicates accurate results.
  - ↓ pH → acidemia.
  - ↑ P_aCO_2 → so this is *primary respiratory acidosis*.
  - Metabolic compensation indicates an acute respiratory acidosis in addition to the chronic respiratory acidosis.
  - AG is normal and HCO_3 is adequately increased → no metabolic disturbances.
  - Conclusion: Acute primary respiratory acidosis on top of a chronic respiratory acidosis. This patient was given a high-flow O_2 (indicated by the high P_aO_2) unnecessarily resulting in retention of CO_2 and severe acute respiratory acidosis. The acute increase in P_aCO_2 resulted in mental deterioration and unresponsiveness.

Case 10

- The patient in the previous case was intubated and mechanically ventilated to protect his airways. A repeat ABG showed pH (7.55), P_aCO_2 (39), P_aO_2 (198), HCO_3 (33), AG (10).

- Interpretation:
  - Applying the Henderson equation indicates accurate results.
  - $\uparrow$ pH $\rightarrow$ alkalemia.
  - The elevated HCO_3 indicates a metabolic alkalosis resulting from overcorrecting the chronic respiratory acidosis. The elevated HCO_3 was primarily a compensatory mechanism for the respiratory acidosis. The resulting metabolic acidosis is sometimes called *posthypercapnic metabolic alkalosis*. The ventilator should have been set to target a normal pH rather than a normal P_aCO_2.

References

1. Bear RA, Dyck RF. Clinical approach to the diagnosis of acid–base disorders. Can Med Assoc J 1979;120:173–182.
2. Kassirer JP, Bleich HL. Rapid estimation of plasma carbon dioxide tension from pH and total carbon dioxide content. N Engl J Med 1965;272:1067.
3. Brackett NC Jr, Cohen JJ, Schwartz WB. Carbon dioxide titration curve of normal man. Effect of increasing degrees of acute hypercapnia on acid–base equilibrium. N Engl J Med 1965;272:6.
4. Schwartz WB, Brackett NC Jr, Cohen JJ. The response of extracellular hydrogen ion concentration to graded degrees of chronic hypercapnia: the physiologic limits of the defense of pH. J Clin Invest 1965;44:291.
5. Arbus GS, Herbert LA, Levesque PR, et al. Characterization and clinical application of the "significance band" for acute respiratory alkalosis. N Engl J Med 1969;280:117.
6. Gennari FJ, Goldstein MB, Schwartz WB. The nature of the renal adaptation to chronic hypocapnia. J Clin Invest 1972;51:1722.
7. Weil JV. Ventilatory control at high altitude. In: Fishman AP, ed. Handbook of Physiology. Section 3: The Respiratory System. American Physiological Society, Bethesda, MD, 1986;703–727.
8. Emmett M, Narins RGL Clinical use of anion gap. Medicine 1977;56: 38–54.
9. Oh MS, Carroll HJ. The anion gap. N Engl J Med 1977;297:814.
10. Lennon EJ, Lemann J Jr. Defense of hydrogen ion concentration in chronic metabolic acidosis. A new evaluation of an old approach. Ann Intern Med 1966;65:265.
11. Albert MD, Sell RB, Winters RW. Quantitative displacement of acid–base equilibrium in metabolic acidosis. Ann Intern Med 1967;66:312.
12. Javaheri S, Kazemi H. Metabolic alkalosis and hypoventilation in humans. Am Rev Respir Dis 1987;136:1101–1116.
13. Fulop M. Hypercapnia in metabolic alkalosis. NY State J Med 1976;76:19.
14. van Ypersele de Strihou C, Frans A. The respiratory response to metabolic alkalosis and acidosis in disease. Clin Sci Mol Med 1973;45:439.
15. Dubose TD. Acid–base disorders. In: Brenner BM, ed. Brenner and Rector's The Kidney, Sixth Edition. WB Saunders, Philadelphia, PA, 2000;925–997.

16. Oliva PB. Severe alveolar hypoventilation in a patient with metabolic alkalosis. Am J Med 1972;52:817.

17. Lifschitz MD, Brasch R, Cuomo AJ, et al. Marked hypercapnia secondary to severe metabolic alkalosis. Ann Intern Med 1972;77:405.

18. Narins RG, Emmett M. Simple and mixed acid–base disorders: a practical approach. Medicine 1980;59:161–187.

19. Fulop M. A guide for predicting arterial CO_2 tension in metabolic acidosis. Am J Nephrol 1997;17:421–424.

20. Goldberg M, Green SB, Moss ML, et al. Computer-based instruction and diagnosis of acid–base disorders: a systematic approach. JAMA 1973;223:266–275.

21. Batlle D, Hizon M, Cohen E, et al: The use of the urinary anion gap in the diagnosis of hyperchloremic metabolic acidosis. N Engl J Med 1988;318:594.

22. Mellemgaard K. The alveolar-arterial oxygen difference: its size and components in normal man. Acta Physiol Scand 1966;67:10.

23. West JB. Respiratory Physiology, the Essentials, Seventh Edition. Lippincott Williams & Wilkins, Philadelphia, PA, 2004.

Chapter 9
Exercise Testing

THE 6-MIN WALK TEST

- The 6MWT is similar to the 12MWT, but the 6MWT is preferred because it is faster, better tolerated, and more standardized.[1,2]
- The 6MWT is a useful tool for both the clinical and research fields. Its main indication is to assess the response of patients with pulmonary or cardiac disorders to certain interventions, e.g., pulmonary hypertension.[1] This test can also be used to assess the functional status and predict mortality and morbidity in such patients. Table 9.1 summarizes the indications and contraindications to 6MWT. The 6MWT is generally safe.[22,27–32] The test should be immediately terminated, however, if the patient develops chest pain, intolerable dyspnea, leg cramps, unstable balance, marked diaphoresis, or pale or ashen appearance.[1]

Technique

- The technique and methodology of 6MWT used for prognostic studies must follow a standardized protocol.
- The 6MWT is best performed in a building with unobstructed level corridors. A distance of 30 m (~100 ft) is considered suitable and the laps are then counted.[1,32–35] Under the supervision of the respiratory therapist, the patient should walk normally, unassisted in carrying portable O_2 cylinder if used.[1,36] The patient is allowed, however, to use any kind of assistance that he/she normally uses for daily activities, e.g., walker. During the test, the patient may be encouraged only by standardized phrases.[1,33,37] The patient is allowed to rest whenever needed.

A. Altalag et al., *Pulmonary Function Tests in Clinical Practice*,
DOI: 10.1007/978-1-84882-231-3_9, © Springer-Verlag London Limited 2009

TABLE 9.1.   Indications & contraindications for the 6MWT

Indications for 6MWT
To assess outcome of therapy (test is done before and after therapy)
   Pulmonary hypertension[1]
   Lung transplantation[3,4]
   Lung resection[5]
   Lung volume reduction surgery[6,7]
   Pulmonary rehabilitation[8,9]
   Drug therapy for COPD[10–12] and heart failure (CHF)[13,14]
To assess functional status in patients with:
   Lung disease (COPD,[15,16] CF,[17,18] and pulmonary hypertension)
   Heart disease (CHF)[19–21]
To predict mortality and morbidity in patients with CHF,[22,23] COPD,[24,25]
   and pulmonary hypertension[4,26]
To assess outcome parameters for research studies

Contraindications[1]
Absolute
   Unstable angina or MI within the past month
Relative
   Resting tachycardia (>120/min)
   Uncontrolled hypertension (systolic >180 and diastolic >100)

A portable pulse oximeter may be used during the test but more important is the reporting of S_pO_2 at the start and the end of the test.[1,38,39]

- The 6MWT is repeated after a sufficient resting period. It is usually reproducible and the largest achieved distance is reported.[1,34]

Interpretation

- Three measurements can be obtained from the 6MWT: the 6-min walk distance (6MWD), the degree of dyspnea and fatigue, and the S_pO_2.[1,36]
- The most important measurement is the 6MWD, which is normally ≥ 580 m in men and 500 m in women.[30] A low 6MWD is nonspecific and nondiagnostic. A low 6MWD may be seen in patients with lung disease, heart disease, and musculoskeletal disease (arthritis) or even in normal subjects who perform a submaximal effort. A significant reduction in the 6MWD, coupled with the appropriate clinical setting is useful to grade the exercise capacity and to evaluate response to therapy and predict the overall outcome. An unexplained reduction of the 6MWD should prompt a search for a possible cause.

- The 6MWD varies significantly among normal individuals. Factors such as age, weight, sex, and height independently influence the 6MWD in healthy adults.[1] Serial measurements of 6MWD in the same patient, to assess disease progression or effect of therapy, given the low intrasubject variability, make the test more useful.
- *The modified Borg scale*, which is a 12-level scale ranging from "no discomfort" to "maximal discomfort," Figure 9.1, may be used to grade the degree of dyspnea that the patient experiences during and at the end of the test.[40]
- S_pO_2 normally is unchanged with exercise. Any drop of >5% usually indicates a respiratory or possibly a cardiac disorder.[41] Artifacts related to signal recording during walking, however, may influence the accuracy of the S_pO_2.[1,38,39]
- Sometimes a walking (exercise) oximetry is done (without measuring the 6MWD) to assess S_pO_2 to determine the need for, or to titrate the level of, supplemental O_2 during exertion. This is often referred to as exercise oximetry and has nothing to do with the 6MWT.

Modified Borg's Scale

0	Nothing at all
0.5	Very, very slight (just noticeable)
1	Very slight
2	Slight (light)
3	Moderate
4	Somewhat severe
5	Severe (heavy)
6	
7	Very severe
8	
9	
10	Very, very severe (Maximal)

FIGURE 9.1. The modified Borg Scale.

CARDIOPULMONARY EXERCISE TESTING

Introduction

- The cardiopulmonary exercise test (CPET) is aimed at assessing the ability of the body organ systems to respond normally during exercise. Exercise normally prompts the delivery of the appropriate amount of O_2 from the external environment to the red blood cells (the function of the pulmonary system). O_2 is then transported to the muscle cells (the function of the cardiovascular system and blood) where oxidative phosphorylation takes place to produce energy (adenosine triphosphate or ATP) (the function of the mitochondria).
- CO_2 should then flow in the opposite direction through the same organ systems until it is exhaled to the external environment. So, these organ systems interact and coordinate their functions together to achieve one goal, the production of energy needed for function, as is illustrated by the Wassermann's gears; Figure 9.2. Therefore, disorders of any of these organ systems result in

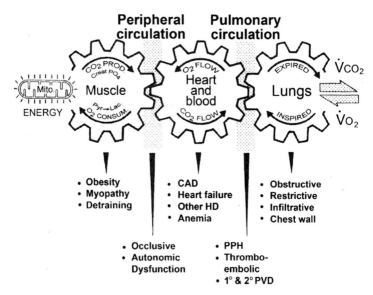

FIGURE 9.2. The Wassermann's gears illustrate the interaction and coordination of the body organ systems to produce energy. Failure of any of the organ systems results in failure of energy production (With permission from Wasserman K, Hansen JE, Sue DY, Stringer WW, Whipp BJ. Principles of Exercise Testing and Interpretation, Fourth Edition. Lippincott Williams & Wilkins, Philadelphia, PA, 2004.).

exercise limitation, i.e., inability to achieve the predicted maximum exercise capacity for a given individual.

- In exercise testing, where subjects are encouraged to achieve their maximum exercise capacity, we aim to achieve two goals: detecting any exercise limitation and identifying the organ system(s) responsible for that limitation.
- The indications and contraindications for exercise testing are listed in Table 9.2.

TABLE 9.2.   Indications and contraindications for CPET

Major indications

To determine exercise capacity/impairment[42]

To identify the cause of exercise limitation[43–52]:

　　If the patient has both cardiac and pulmonary diseases and unsure which is most responsible for the exercise limitation

　　If no cause is apparent for exercise limitation after full evaluation

Assessment of exercise capacity if resting data do not explain symptoms[42,52]

Assessment of therapy selection and response (pulmonary rehabilitation,[53–55] lung resection,[56–58] lung transplantation,[59,60] cardiac transplantation,[44,61,62] medical therapy for lung diseases such as COPD,[63–68] pulmonary hypertension,[69–72] ILD,[73,74] and CF[75,76])

Evaluation for impairment/disability[77–82]

Other indications

Diagnosis of exercise-induced asthma[83–87]

Identification of gas-exchange abnormalities[42,44]

Titration of supplemental O_2 rate during exercise[64,88–93]

Absolute contraindications[91,94,95]

Active cardiac disease (acute MI, unstable angina, active arrhythmias, uncontrolled CHF, severe aortic stenosis, aortic dissection, endocarditis, myocarditis, pericarditis)

Active pulmonary disease (uncontrolled asthma, respiratory failure, pulmonary edema, acute PE or DVT)

Hemodynamic instability or acute noncardiopulmonary disease affecting exercise performance (infection, thyroid disease)

Relative contraindications[42,72]

Uncontrolled systemic (systolic >200 mmHg; diastolic >120 mmHg) or pulmonary hypertension

Hypertrophic obstructive cardiomyopathy

Significant left main coronary artery stenosis (without acute symptoms)

Others (moderate stenotic valvular heart disease, advanced pregnancy, electrolyte abnormalities, orthopedic impairment)

Equipment

- A *cycle ergometer* or a treadmill
  - Represents a way to apply a controlled quantifiable workload that can be steadily increased.
  - An ergometer is generally preferred over a treadmill because of the following:
    (a) Ergometer is associated with less body movements, which produce fewer artifacts in the recorded data.[42,52]
    (b) A more linear and quantifiable workload can be achieved by the ergometer.[42,44,52]
    (c) Ergometer is less expensive and occupies less space.[42]
- Respiratory system monitors:
  - *Gas analyzers*: measure the amounts of the exhaled O_2 and CO_2 throughout exercise, from which many exercise parameters are derived.[42,96]
  - *Airflow or volume recording device*: is used to measure ventilation during exercise, from which other useful data can be derived.[42]
  - *Pulse oximeter*: is used to record S_pO_2 throughout exercise (its function is different from the gas analyzer that measures the amount of exhaled O_2).[97–99]
  - More invasive methods can be used *(arterial line)* to monitor the arterial blood gases (ABG for P_aO_2 and bicarbonate) and lactate. These measurements are not routinely needed.[100]
  - *The modified Borg scale chart*: can be used to grade the degree of discomfort the patient experiences in terms of breathlessness and leg fatigue during different stages of exercise; Figure 9.1.[101] Breathlessness and leg fatigue are the two major symptoms that limit exercise.[102–104]
- Cardiovascular monitors:
  - Include baseline and continuous *ECG monitoring* throughout exercise, which monitors the heart rate (HR) and aids in detecting arrhythmias and ischemia.[105,106]
  - Continuous (through an arterial line)[42,107,108] or, more commonly, intermittent (cuff system)[106]*blood pressure (BP) monitoring* is also done.

Technique

- The CPET equipment must be calibrated before use to meet strict quality control parameters in order to ensure accurate measurements.[42,106,109–115]
- The technique involves asking the patient to pedal the cycle ergometer at a fixed speed with a progressive increase in the

resistance to pedaling (work rate or WR). The patient is connected, throughout the test, to a number of instruments, namely, a mouthpiece for gas collection and flow and volume measurements, ECG monitor, pulse oximeter, and a blood pressure cuff. These instruments will feed data to a computer with software that can plot the results in both a graphic and numeric format. The test is terminated once any of the factors listed in Table 9.3 arise. ABG may then be withdrawn (if arterial line is placed) and a recovery period starts.

- Continuous supervision by a properly trained technologist and a physician is mandatory throughout exercise.[42]

O_2 Uptake, Major Concepts

- Understanding O_2 uptake is the window to understanding the body's physiological changes in response to exercise. This section discusses the major concepts of $\dot{V}O_2$.

Definitions

- $\dot{V}O_2$ (O_2 uptake):
  - Is the amount of O_2 in liters that the body consumes per minute (liters/minute).
  - $\dot{V}O_2$ (in L/min) represents the internal metabolic work and is directly proportional to the external WR (in watts) applied through the cycle ergometer or treadmill; that is why $\dot{V}O_2$ is considered equivalent to WR. Therefore, whenever you encounter "$\dot{V}O_2$" remember that it represents WR used during the test.[42]
- Maximum $\dot{V}O_2$ ($\dot{V}O_2$ max) (L/min):

TABLE 9.3. Indications for termination of exercise testing[42, 44, 52, 116–119]

Severe dyspnea or fatigue at peak exercise
Ventilatory limitation or severe symptomatic desaturation ($S_pO_2 \leq 80\%$)
Reaching a plateau of $\dot{V}O_2$ vs. WR curve (but not reaching the predicted max HR[42]); patients may be encouraged to continue exercising if they can.
Significant degree of lactic acidosis → either HCO_3 ↓ by 5 meq/L or ↑ in RER to 1.15[120]
Significant ECG changes (ischemia, arrhythmias, high-grade AV blocks)
BP instability (systolic BP of >250 mmHg or dropping by >20 mmHg from the highest value during CPET; diastolic BP of >120 mmHg)
Signs and symptoms of cardiovascular, respiratory or CNS instability (sudden pallor, loss of coordination, mental confusion, dizziness, syncope, respiratory failure)

- Is the maximum achievable $\dot{V}O_2$ (workload). $\dot{V}O_2$ max can be detected when the $\dot{V}O_2$ plateaus in relation to the external workload (WR), indicating that no further increase in $\dot{V}O_2$ can be achieved despite increasing WR; Figure 9.11c.[42,119] $\dot{V}O_2$ max represents the maximum exercise capacity for a given subject and is an indication for exercise termination, see Table 9.3.
- Measured peak $\dot{V}O_2$ (L/min):
  - Is the highest $\dot{V}O_2$ that a subject actually achieves during CPET.
- Predicted peak $\dot{V}O_2$ (L/min):
  - Is the highest $\dot{V}O_2$ (workload) that a subject is expected to achieve.
  - It is determined by the patient's age, sex, and body size.[42,89,121]
  - In normal subjects, the measured peak $\dot{V}O_2$ usually equals predicted peak $\dot{V}O_2$ while in patients with heart or lung disease the measured peak $\dot{V}O_2$ is often less than predicted peak $\dot{V}O_2$.
- $\dot{V}O_2$/kg (ml/min/kg):
  - Is the O_2 consumption in milliliters/minute corrected for the body weight in kg. It is particularly useful in interpreting the test in obese individuals.

Factors Determining $\dot{V}O_2$

- These factors can be acquired from the *Fick equation*,[122] which can be written as follows (for details see Table 9.4):

$$\dot{V}O_2 = SV \times HR \times (1.34) \times Hgb \times (S_aO_2 - S_{\bar{v}}O_2).$$

TABLE 9.4. Fick equation[122]

It states that the cardiac output equals the rate of O_2 uptake divided by the difference in the arterial and mixed venous O_2 content:

$$C.O. = \dot{V}O_2/C_aO_2 - C_{\bar{v}}O_2$$

$$SO : \dot{V}O_2 = C.O. \times (C_aO_2 - C_{\bar{v}}O_2)$$

Because C.O. = SV × HR, then:

$$\dot{V}O_2 = SV \times HR \times (C_aO_2 - C_{\bar{v}}O_2)$$

Because: $(C_aO_2 - C_{\bar{v}}O_2) = (1.34) \times Hgb \times (S_aO_2 - S_{\bar{v}}O_2) + [(0.003) \times (P_aO_2 - P_{\bar{v}}O_2)]$ and because: $[(0.003) \times (P_aO_2 - P_{\bar{v}}O_2)]$ is negligible, then the final equation can be written as follows:

$\dot{V}O_2 = SV \times HR \times (1.34) \times Hgb \times (S_aO_2 - S_{\bar{v}}O_2)$, where SV is the stroke volume, HR is the heart rate, Hgb is the hemoglobin, S_aO_2 is the arterial O_2 saturation, and $S_{\bar{v}}O_2$ is the mixed venous O_2 saturation

- From this equation, the factors that determine $\dot{V}O_2$ are HR, SV, Hgb, and the difference between the arterial and mixed venous O_2 content (i.e., the ability of muscle cells to extract O_2 from the blood). During exercise, these factors progressively increase in response to the increased WR, with the exception of Hgb. As an example, at peak exercise, the amount of O_2 extracted from the blood ($S_aO_2 - S_{\bar{v}}O_2$) is threefold higher than at the start of exercise.[42,44] Similarly, C.O. can increase by up to fourfold at peak exercise by increasing HR and SV.[123]
- Conditions that affect any of these factors will necessarily affect $\dot{V}O_2$ and hence the exercise capacity:
  - Patients with a cardiac disease (like cardiomyopathy) cannot increase their SV appropriately in response to exercise resulting in exercise limitation. In highly trained athletes, however, there is an augmented increase in SV in response to exercise resulting in a supranormal exercise capacity; Figure 9.5.[124]
  - Patients with chronotropic disorders (e.g., pacemaker patients with fixed HR or patients on β-blockers) cannot increase their HR appropriately with exercise; hence, they are exercise limited.
  - Patients with anemia (or carboxy-hemoglobinemia) may have low exercise capacity because of low O_2 carrying capacity.
  - Patients with muscle disease that impairs O_2 extraction and utilization (e.g., mitochondrial disease) will have exercise limitation.

Assessing the Cardiovascular System

$\dot{V}O_2$ Relationship with the Cardiac Output Components

- As discussed earlier, the two components determining C.O. are HR and SV; C.O. = SV × HR.
- During exercise, there is a near linear increase in C.O. with increasing WR ($\dot{V}O_2$), initially accomplished by increases in both SV and HR (to a lesser extent). Then, SV plateaus, at which time HR increases more rapidly; Figure 9.3.[44]
- Normally we are exercise-limited by our heart, that is, we stop exercising when we achieve our maximum HR.[125–127] So, it is important to determine the predicted maximum HR so that we can define our cardiac limits to exercise.
- The predicted maximum HR depends on the age and can be derived from different formulae:
  - Max HR = 220 – age[89] *or* Max HR = 210 – (0.65 × age).[128]

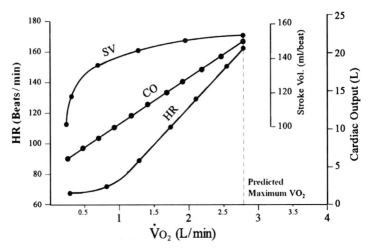

FIGURE 9.3. The relationship between $\dot{V}O_2$ and C.O. components. SV increases first then when it plateaus, HR increases more rapidly. This maintains a linear increase in C.O.

- The HR can be easily measured during exercise, while the SV generally requires a more invasive method (e.g., cardiac catheterization). A search for a noninvasive method to estimate SV resulted in the concept of the "O_2 pulse."

O_2 Pulse ($\dot{V}O_2$/HR)

- Is defined as the O_2 uptake or consumption (in L/min) for each cardiac cycle, i.e., $\dot{V}O_2$ divided by the HR. The Fick equation can then be rearranged to calculate O_2 pulse:

$$O_2 \text{ pulse or } \dot{V}O_2 / HR = SV \times 1.34 \times Hgb \times (S_aO_2 - S_{\bar{v}}O_2).$$

- Assuming that the variables in the right side of this equation are constant [Hgb and $(S_aO_2 - S_{\bar{v}}O_2)$], then O_2 pulse becomes equivalent to SV. That is why, O_2 pulse is used by some as a noninvasive surrogate marker for SV in exercise test interpretation.[89,91] When O_2 pulse is plotted against $\dot{V}O_2$, it produces a curve comparable to SV curve; Figure 9.3. The assumption that the a–$\bar{v}$ O_2 saturation difference is constant is not always true. The O_2 pulse is a more qualitative assessment of SV and must be viewed in this context for interpretation.

- When O_2 pulse (SV) fails to increase appropriately with exercise, it may indicate cardiac disease, e.g., cardiomyopathy, as discussed earlier. As a result, the body will compensate by increasing HR to maintain an appropriate increase in C.O., which is required to continue exercising. The patient will end up reaching the maximum HR much earlier than expected, resulting in premature termination of exercise (i.e., a low peak $\dot{V}O_2$); see Figures 9.4 and 9.5.[129] A low O_2 pulse can also be seen in deconditioning.[42]
- By looking at the curves in Figure 9.4, we can make two comments:
  - There is a significant reduction in peak $\dot{V}O_2$ (i.e., exercise limitation).
  - The steep increase in HR with minimal increase in O_2 pulse (SV) indicates a cardiovascular origin of exercise limitation.
- Aerobic training, however, results in a higher SV for a given workload, thus a lower HR. A higher $\dot{V}O_2$ therefore, can be achieved (e.g., elite athletes may more than double their peak $\dot{V}O_2$); Figure 9.5.[130]

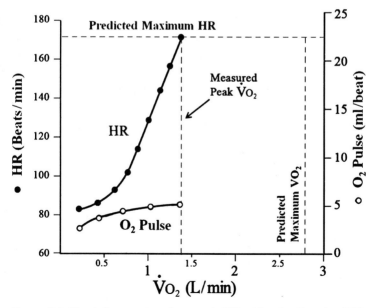

FIGURE 9.4. Heart disease, steep increase in HR with a flat O_2 pulse (SV); peak $\dot{V}O_2$ is reduced.

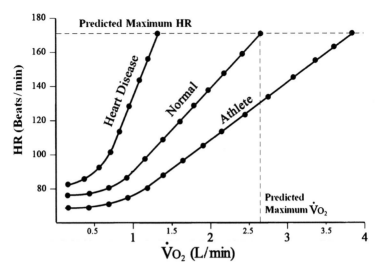

FIGURE 9.5. HR reaches its peak early in heart disease and late in aerobic training resulting in a significant difference in peak $\dot{V}O_2$ in the two conditions.

- If peak exercise is reached before reaching the maximum HR, this is referred to as HR reserve:

  HR reserve = Pred. HR max – achieved HR at peak $\dot{V}O_2$.

- HR reserve is increased in patients with pulmonary disease and those who cannot reach their peak exercise for other reasons (e.g., volitional, muscle fatigue).

Definition of Other Exercise Parameters

- $\dot{V}CO_2$: is the amount of CO_2 produced by the body per minute (L/min).
- *Respiratory quotient (RQ):* is the amount of CO_2 the body produces for each liter (mole) of O_2 it consumes, at the tissue level. Normally, at rest, we produce ~0.8 mole of CO_2 for each mole of O_2 we consume (RQ = 0.8), but this increases with exercise as will be discussed.
- *Respiratory exchange ratio (RER):* is the amount of CO_2 produced per liter of O_2 consumed as measured from the exhaled air at the mouth ($\dot{V}CO_2/\dot{V}O_2$). At steady state, RER equals RQ

allowing RER to be used as a rough index of RQ given the difficulty of measuring the later.[42]

- $\dot{V}E$ *(minute ventilation)*: is the volume of air we breathe per minute. $\dot{V}E$ is the product of tidal volume (V_T) and respiratory rate (RR):

$$\dot{V}E = \dot{V}_T \times RR.$$

- $P_{ET}O_2$: is the end-tidal O_2 tension as measured from the exhaled air.
- $P_{ET}CO_2$: is the end-tidal CO_2 tension as measured from the exhaled air.
- *Ventilatory equivalent for $\dot{V}O_2$ i.e., ($\dot{V}E/\dot{V}O_2$)*: is the amount of $\dot{V}E$ for a given level of $\dot{V}O_2$ (WR).
- *Ventilatory equivalent for $\dot{V}CO_2$, i.e., ($\dot{V}E/\dot{V}CO_2$)*: is the amount of $\dot{V}E$ at a given level of $\dot{V}CO_2$.

Anaerobic Threshold (AT)

- Is defined as the $\dot{V}O_2$ (in L/min) at which there is substantial transition to anaerobic metabolism to produce extra energy (ATP). This is aimed at supplementing aerobic metabolism, which becomes insufficient at higher levels of exercise (in healthy subjects AT takes place at ~45–60% of predicted peak $\dot{V}O_2$[85,86]).
- AT is called anaerobic because this process is O_2 independent. At the same time, it results in the production of lactic acid, which when accumulating, contributes to muscle fatigue leading to termination of exercise. This is why AT is sometimes called *lactate threshold*.[131,132] The body buffers the rising levels of lactic acid in the blood with bicarbonate to stabilize the pH:

$$Lactate^- + H^+ + HCO_3^- \rightarrow H_2CO_3 \rightarrow H_2O + CO_2.$$

- As a result, extra CO_2 is produced, unrelated to O_2 consumed ($\dot{V}O_2$) resulting in the rise of RER during exercise, which often exceeds 1 (i.e., more CO_2 is produced than the O_2 consumed). Because of this accelerated rise in CO_2 ($\dot{V}CO_2$) at AT, the respiratory system responds by eliminating the extra CO_2, resulting in a rise in $\dot{V}E$ out of proportion to $\dot{V}O_2$ if they are plotted against each other; Figure 9.6a. The point at which the slope of $\dot{V}E$ curve changes is called the inflection point and corresponds to AT; Figure 9.6a.

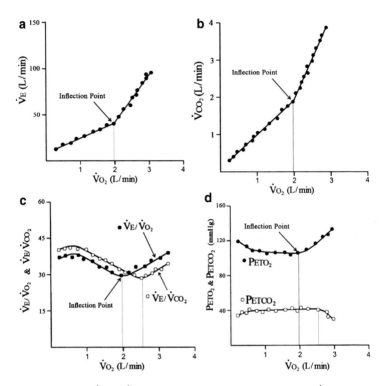

FIGURE 9.6. (a) $\dot{V}E$ vs $\dot{V}O_2$ curve showing a steady increase in $\dot{V}E$, then at AT it inflects upward. (b) $\dot{V}CO_2$ vs. $\dot{V}O_2$ curve. (c) $\dot{V}E/\dot{V}O_2$ vs. $\dot{V}O_2$ curve and $\dot{V}E/\dot{V}CO_2$ vs. $\dot{V}O_2$ curve. (d) $P_{ET}O_2$ vs. $\dot{V}O_2$ curve and $P_{ET}CO_2$ vs. $\dot{V}O_2$ curve.

- Methods to identify AT include the following:
  - $\dot{V}E$ vs. $\dot{V}O_2$ curve, as discussed earlier; Figure 9.6a.
  - $\dot{V}CO_2$ vs. $\dot{V}O_2$ curve; Figure 9.6b. As at AT, $\dot{V}CO_2$ rises faster because of the increased CO_2 production; this is called the $\dot{V}$-slope.[163]
  - Ventilatory equivalents for $\dot{V}O_2$ and $\dot{V}CO_2$ i.e., ($\dot{V}E/\dot{V}O_2$ and $\dot{V}E/\dot{V}CO_2$) vs. $\dot{V}O_2$ curve; Figure 9.6c[42]:
    (a) With exercise, $\dot{V}E/\dot{V}O_2$ drops steadily as the increase in $\dot{V}O_2$ (denominator) exceeds the increase in $\dot{V}E$ (numera-

tor), until AT is reached when the ($\dot{V}E/\dot{V}O_2$) inflects upward due to the disproportionate increase in $\dot{V}E$ compared with that in $\dot{V}O_2$.

(b) This inflection point may be clearer in this curve than in the $\dot{V}E$ vs. $\dot{V}O_2$ curve, as the $\dot{V}E/\dot{V}O_2$ vs. $\dot{V}O_2$ plot changes direction from downward to upward.

(c) On the other hand, the ventilatory equivalent for $\dot{V}CO_2$ ($\dot{V}E/\dot{V}CO_2$) continues to decrease after $\dot{V}E/\dot{V}O_2$ inflection point (AT) is reached, as, at AT, both the denominator ($\dot{V}CO_2$) and numerator ($\dot{V}E$) increase proportionately initially. This downward slope of $\dot{V}E/\dot{V}CO_2$ vs. $\dot{V}O_2$ curve continues beyond AT until $\dot{V}E$ disproportionately increases as a compensation when a frank metabolic acidosis develops, at which point the curve changes direction upward; Figure 9.6c.[42]

- $P_{ET}O_2$ and $P_{ET}CO_2$ vs. $\dot{V}O_2$ curve; Figure 9.6d:

(a) The expired O_2 tension remains stable during exercise but inflects upward at AT in response to the increased $\dot{V}E$.

(b) $P_{ET}CO_2$ similarly remains stable at and beyond AT for some time before deflecting downward in response to the disproportionate increase in $\dot{V}E$ when a frank metabolic acidosis develops.[42]

- AT can also be determined invasively by serial measurements of lactate or bicarbonate (ABG) during exercise. At AT, lactate rises and bicarbonate drops (to buffer the lactic acid) in the same ratio (they are equimolar).[133,134] So, if lactate or HCO_3^- is plotted against $\dot{V}O_2$, then the point at which the lactate starts rising or HCO_3^- starts dropping corresponds to the AT; Figure 9.7.[42,135,136]

• The AT is determined predominantly by the cardiovascular system. If C.O. does not increase appropriately during exercise, it will result in impaired O_2 delivery to the muscles and a faster transition to anaerobic metabolism. This means that in cardiovascular disease, the AT is generally low (<40% of peak $\dot{V}O_2$) and contributes to exercise limitation because of muscle fatigue (accumulation of lactate). Other causes of reduced AT include deconditioning, reduction in O_2 carrying capacity, and muscle oxidative disorders.[42] In respiratory disease, the AT is either normal, not reached[137,138] or indeterminate[139] as the patient is usually limited by ventilatory constraints.

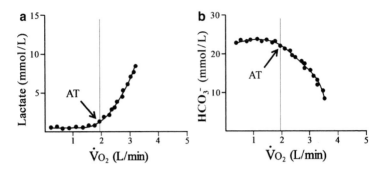

FIGURE 9.7. At AT, HCO_3 starts to drop and lactate starts to rise.

Blood Pressure Response[42,140]

- BP is another parameter used to assess cardiovascular function. Normally, the systolic BP increases with exercise because of increased C.O., and the diastolic BP remains unchanged or drops slightly because of decreased systemic vascular resistance in response to vasodilatation in the exercising muscles.
- An excessive rise in BP (e.g., systolic >220 mmHg; diastolic >100 mmHg) during exercise suggests abnormal sympathetic BP control, but may also be seen in patients with known resting hypertension.
- Failure of BP to rise with exercise suggests a cardiac disorder or abnormal sympathetic control of BP.
- A drop of BP with exercise should prompt exercise termination as it indicates either a serious cardiac disorder (CHF, aortic stenosis, or ischemia) or circulatory disorder (pulmonary vascular disease or central pulmonary venous obstruction).

Assessing the Respiratory System

The respiratory system is assessed as two components: the ventilatory component and the gas-exchange component.

Ventilatory Component

Definitions

- *Maximal voluntary ventilation (MVV)*

– Is the maximum minute ventilation that a subject can achieve. It is used as an estimation of the predicted $\dot{V}E$ at peak exercise (predicted $\dot{V}E$ max). It can be determined mathematically as follows:

(a) *Calculated MVV*: derived from the patient's FEV_1,[53,141–145] which is the technique used by most clinical exercise laboratories*,†,††:

$$MVV = FEV_1(L) \times 40.$$

(b) *Predicted MVV* is calculated from the patient's height, sex, and age by multiplying the predicted (not measured) FEV_1 by 40.* Therefore, in respiratory disease, the calculated MVV will often be less than the patient's predicted MVV.

- $\dot{V}E$ *max*: is the maximum $\dot{V}E$ that the patient achieves during CPET.
- *Ventilatory reserve* = Predicted – measured $\dot{V}E$ max, i.e., = MVV – $\dot{V}E$ max.[44,52,89]
- *Breathing reserve (another way of expressing ventilatory reserve)* = measured/predicted $\dot{V}E$ max, i.e.,
  = $\dot{V}Emax/MVV$.[44,52,89]

$\dot{V}E$, Major Concepts

- The components of $\dot{V}E$ are RR and V_T:

$$\dot{V}E = RR \times V_T$$

- During exercise, the V_T increases initially rapidly and then plateaus, at which point the RR increases maintaining a linear increase in $\dot{V}E$; Figure 9.8.[130,146,147]
- Unlike HR, the maximum RR (50/min) is not reached normally at peak exercise ($\dot{V}O_2$), allowing for some reserve in $\dot{V}E$

---

* Some laboratories use 35 instead of 40 as the conversion factor; the equation will then be: $MVV = FEV_1 \times 35$.

†*Measured MVV*: is determined in the lab by measuring the patient's ventilation over 12 s during a maximal effort, then the result is extrapolated to 1 min by multiplying by 5; see Chapter 5, Figure 5.1. If both measured and calculated MVV are done (which is unusual), the higher of the two is reported as the predicted $\dot{V}E$ max.

†† Calculated MVV is often referred to in the final CPET as the predicted $\dot{V}E$ max

(~30–40% of the predicted V̇Emax). This can be expressed as either ventilatory or breathing reserve; see earlier definitions.

- This means that if V̇E max is achieved during exercise, then the patient is generally exercise-limited by ventilatory parameters, and stops exercise because of dyspnea; Figure 9.9.
- Elite athletes may achieve their V̇E max (MVV) during exercise, but they reach their V̇E max at a higher than predicted V̇O$_2$; Figure 9.9. This may indicate that elite athletes have such well-conditioned oxygen delivery from the lungs to the working muscle that they reach their V̇E max and may thus be exercise limited by their lungs!
- Ventilatory limitation may also occur when dynamic hyperinflation is recognized in the tidal flow–volume loops recorded during exercise. Dynamic hyperinflation leads to a progressive rise in FRC during exercise. This will lead to a left shift of the tidal flow–volume loops with the end-inspiratory lung volume approaching TLC and the tidal expiratory flow reaching or approaching the maximal expiratory envelope. This flow limitation and mechanical constraint increase the work of breathing and limit exercise capacity.[64,148–151] Dynamic hyperinflation is probably the main cause of breathlessness in patients with COPD (emphysema); Figure 9.10.

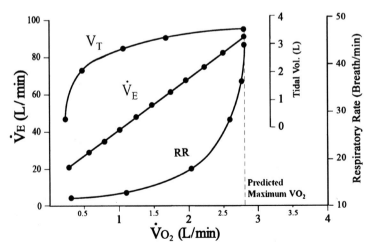

FIGURE 9.8. Behavior of V_T and RR during exercise is similar to SV and HR. Note that V̇E and V̇O$_2$ maintain a linear relationship.

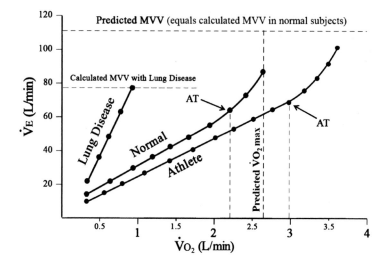

FIGURE 9.9. Patients with lung disease reach their predicted $\dot{V}E$ max early, notice that the calculated MVV (i.e. the predicted $\dot{V}E$ max) is less than the predicted MVV in patients with lung disease. Elite athletes may approach their predicted MVV with a supranormal $\dot{V}O_2$.

- P_aCO_2 and $P_{ET}CO_2$ normally remain stable until AT is reached, when they start to decrease due to the increased $\dot{V}E$. In some ventilatory disorders, however, both P_aCO_2 and $P_{ET}CO_2$ can increase due to a relative hypoventilation. Although P_aCO_2 and $P_{ET}CO_2$ may be used to assess ventilatory function, they are considered also useful in assessing gas-exchange function as will be explained later.

Gas-Exchange Component

This is assessed by three ways: dead space fraction, ABG, and RQ.

Dead Space Fraction

- At rest, V_T is normally ~450 ml, one-third of which (150 ml) is wasted in the anatomic and physiologic dead spaces (dead space volume, V_D). The other two-thirds reach the gas-exchange units and are referred to as the alveolar volume (V_A), so:

$$V_T = V_D + V_A.$$

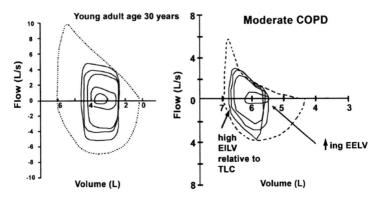

FIGURE 9.10. Normally, tidal flow–volume loops expand from both directions during exercise. In emphysema, the decreased expiratory time (because of increased RR during exercise) results in more air-trapping and increases the FRC, shifting the tidal FV curves to the left, a phenomenon called *dynamic hyperinflation*. (With permission from ATS/ACCP Statement on Cardiopulmonary Exercise Testing. Am J Respir Crit Care Med 2003;167:211–277.).

- Similarly, this equation can be applied to the $\dot{V}$E:

$$\dot{V}_E = \dot{V}_D + \dot{V}_A.$$

- Dead space fraction (V_D/V_T) is then the dead space volume expressed as a fraction of V_T. It similarly equals $\dot{V}_D/\dot{V}_E$.
- At rest, dead space fraction is 150 ml/450 ml, which equals 1/3, as discussed. During exercise, however, V_T increases to 800 ml or more[‡] with a relatively constant dead space volume[§], resulting in a reduction of dead space fraction from ~1/3 to ~1/5, which improves gas exchange.[52]
- At rest, the upper lobes of the lungs are not as well perfused as the bases but with exercise, perfusion improves to the upper

---

[‡]V_T can reach as high as 2.5 L with exercise.

[§]In reality V_D does not remain constant with exercise; it increases slightly and may reach 200 ml. This is due to a number of factors including exercise-induced bronchodilatation and distension of airways related to the increased lung volumes.[152]

lobes (because of increased blood flow) resulting in a more even $\dot{V}/Q$ distribution and hence better gas exchange.[52]

- In summary, we normally improve our gas exchange during exercise by increasing alveolar ventilation more than dead space and improving overall $\dot{V}/Q$ matching.

- On the other hand, diseases that interfere with dead space fraction during exercise result in an inefficient gas-exchange process and can contribute to premature termination of exercise. Lung fibrosis is an example, where the stiff small lungs are incapable of increasing the V_T appropriately in response to exercise. So, V_D/V_T remains unchanged or does not decrease as expected with exercise as the excessive increase in RR at a low V_T increases the volume of wasted ventilation (dead space).

- Estimating V_D/V_T allows for detection of such diseases. This may be done in two ways:

  – V_D/V_T can be measured from *the dead space equation*:[153,¶]

  $$V_D/V_T = (P_aCO_2 - P_{\bar{E}}CO_2)/P_aCO_2,$$

  where $P_{\bar{E}}CO_2$ is the mixed expired CO_2 measured in exhaled samples. The smaller the difference between P_aCO_2 and $P_{\bar{E}}CO_2$ (i.e., the higher the $P_{\bar{E}}CO_2$), the lower the V_D/V_T, that is, the more efficient the ventilation is. To measure this parameter noninvasively $P_{ET}CO_2$ is substituted for P_aCO_2.

  – The other way is using *the mass balance equation* that can be rearranged as follows[52]:

  $$\frac{\dot{V}E}{\dot{V}CO_2} = K \times \frac{1}{P_aCO_2\left[1-\left(V_D/V_T\right)\right]}.$$

  – From this equation, the ventilatory equivalent for $\dot{V}CO_2$ ($\dot{V}E/\dot{V}CO_2$) can be used as a noninvasive surrogate marker for the dead space fraction (V_D/V_T) if P_aCO_2 remains constant. This assumption can be applied near or at the AT, but not beyond that, when P_aCO_2 drops in response to increased $\dot{V}E$ (to compensate for the lactic acidosis).

¶This equation is derived from Bohr's law, which states that the product of volume and concentration is the same under constant temperature.

Other Methods for Assessing Gas Exchange

- A–a gradient ($P_{(A-a)}O_2$)
  - At rest, $P_{(A-a)}O_2$ is normally <10 mmHg and increases with exercise to >20 mmHg, as P_AO_2 normally increases with exercise and P_aO_2 remains normal. However, any increase in $P_{(A-a)}O_2$ of >35 mmHg with exercise is considered abnormal and indicates a gas-exchange abnormality.[42,154,155]
  - $P_{(A-a)}O_2$ can be calculated from *the alveolar gas equation* as follows (see Chapter 8 for details):

$$P_{(A-a)}O_2 = [P_IO_2 - \frac{P_aCO_2}{RQ}] - P_aO_2.$$

  - RQ is substituted for by RER that is measured simultaneously with P_aO_2 and P_aCO_2 during and at the end of exercise.
- S_pO_2 (pulse oximetry) or S_aO_2 (ABG)
  - S_pO_2 is the standard measure of oxygenation used during exercise testing. It may be less accurate than S_aO_2 particularly at low levels and can be prone to artifact.[156,157] Both S_pO_2 and S_aO_2 should remain normal and stable with exercise. Any drop of ≥5% indicates a gas-exchange abnormality.[94,158] A significant symptomatic desaturation (<80%) during exercise indicates a significant gas-exchange disorder and should prompt exercise cessation; see Table 9.3.
- P_aO_2
  - Remains stable or increases slightly with exercise. A drop in P_aO_2 indicates a gas-exchange abnormality.
- RER should not exceed 1.3 at peak exercise. If so, it indicates a gas-exchange abnormality. This is a useful measurement to determine if peak exercise is truly achieved (RER of ≥1.15 generally indicates maximal effort).[120]
- P_aCO_2 and $P_{ET}CO_2$ are increased in gas-exchange disorders.

Approach to Exercise Test Interpretation

In interpreting any cardiopulmonary exercise study, you have to apply a structured approach (Table 9.5 shows one suggestion). The following are the major steps in interpreting such studies:

Maximal Effort

Determine whether a truly maximal effort was achieved. A maximal effort is achieved if one or more of the factors listed in Table 9.6 is

TABLE 9.5. Suggested steps in reading exercise testing

Determine:
- The indication for CPET.
- Determine the type of exercise tool used (usually cycle ergometer)
- Report the reason for exercise termination (dyspnea, leg discomfort, fatigue)
- Report the Borg scoring for dyspnea and leg discomfort at exercise termination.

Examine the base-line spirometry and maximal flow volume loop.

Determine whether a truly maximal effort was achieved; Table 9.5.

Determine whether exercise capacity is normal:
- Determine the peak $\dot{V}O_2$ (should be >83% predicted), this can be done numerically or through $\dot{V}O_2$ vs. WR curve.
- Determine the maximum WR achieved (>80% predicted).
- Determine the severity of exercise limitation, which can be graded according to $\dot{V}O_2$ max. as mild (60–83% pred.), moderate (40–60% pred.), and severe (<40% pred.).

Examine the cardiovascular response:
- Examine HR response (remember that max HR should be achieved at peak exercise).
- HR max (should be >90% of predicted)
- Calculate HR reserve = predicted – achieved HR (normal is ±15)
- HR curve (should be along the predicted curve)
- Examine O_2 pulse at peak $\dot{V}O_2$
- Determine the value of O_2 pulse at peak exercise (>80% predicted)
- O_2 pulse curve should run along the predicted curve
- Determine AT (>40% predicted $\dot{V}O_2$); graphically identify AT from: $\dot{V}E$, $\dot{V}CO_2$, $\dot{V}E/\dot{V}O_2$ and $P_{ET}O_2$ curves.
- Examine $\dot{V}O_2$ vs. WR curve; it should run along the predicted curve.
- Report the BP (normally: 205 ± 25 over 100 ± 10; i.e. ↑ systolic and pulse pressures)
- Examine the ECG for arrhythmia and/or ischemia

Examine the ventilatory response:
- Determine $\dot{V}E$ max (<70% of predicted MVV)
- Compare the calculated MVV to the predicted MVV.
  - Examine $\dot{V}E$ curve (should be along the predicted curve and should not reach MVV)
  - Determine $\dot{V}E$ (ventilatory) reserve = calculated MVV – $\dot{V}E$ max (>15)
  - Determine the breathing reserve = $\dot{V}E$ max/calculated MVV (0.72 ± 0.15)
- RR max (<50)
- Examine tidal FV loops for dynamic hyperinflation.

Examine the gas-exchange response:
- Examine the dead space fraction:
  - V_D/V_T normally decreases with exercise
  - Determine $\dot{V}E/\dot{V}CO_2$ at AT (<34) – a surrogate marker for V_D fraction
  - Determine $\dot{V}E/\dot{V}O_2$ at AT (<31)
- Check $P_{ET}CO_2$ (and P_aCO_2) at peak exercise (it normally decreases)

(continued)

Table 9.5 (continued)

Determine RER at peak $\dot{V}O_2$ (1.1–1.3)
Determine S_pO_2 (more accurately S_aO_2) at peak $\dot{V}O_2$ (it should not drop by >5%)
ABG at the end of exercise
  P_aO_2 is unchanged normally with exercise
  $P_{(A-a)}O_2$ increases slightly but should not exceed 35 mmHg.
Finally, the conclusion

Table 9.6. Factors suggesting a maximal effort[42,119,120]

Achieving predicted peak $\dot{V}O_2$ and/or a plateau is observed in $\dot{V}O_2$ vs. WR curve.
Achieving predicted maximum WR.
Achieving predicted maximum HR.
$\dot{V}E$ max. approaching or exceeding the calculated MVV.
RER of ≥1.15.
Patient exhaustion with a Borg scale rating of 9–10.

(are) present. Lack of these factors indicates a submaximal effort, which may limit the usefulness of the CPET.

Exercise Capacity

Determine whether the exercise capacity is normal by checking the peak $\dot{V}O_2$, WR, and their relationship:

- Peak $\dot{V}O_2$ should be more than 83% of the predicted peak $\dot{V}O_2$ ($\dot{V}O_2$ max). If peak $\dot{V}O_2$ is normal, then you are likely to be dealing with a normal subject. If peak $\dot{V}O_2$ is reduced, then you need to determine the cause, which could be cardiac disease, pulmonary disease, neuromuscular disease, deconditioning, reduced oxygen carrying capacity, or submaximal effort. The degree of impairment of exercise capacity is graded into mild, moderate, and severe depending on peak $\dot{V}O_2$ (e.g., peak $\dot{V}O_2$ of 60–83% pred. is mild, 40–60% pred. is moderate, and <40% pred. is severe).
- Achieving the predicted WR (in watts) also indicates a normal exercise capacity, while failure to achieve the predicted WR indicates a decreased exercise capacity.
- Graphically, looking at $\dot{V}O_2$ vs. WR curve serves the same purpose. If the curve reaches the predicted peak $\dot{V}O_2$, then the exercise capacity is normal; Figure 9.11a. A subnormal exercise capacity is indicated when the curve does not reach the predicted peak $\dot{V}O_2$, with or without an early plateau; Figure 9.11b, c.

Cardiovascular System

Determine whether the cardiovascular response to exercise is normal by looking at the HR max, O_2 pulse, the onset of AT, $\dot{V}O_2$ vs. WR curve, BP, and ECG.

• The predicted HR max is reached at the predicted peak $\dot{V}O_2$ in normal subjects (Figure 9.12a), but is reached prematurely in patients with heart disease. This is because these patients cannot increase their stroke volume (SV) appropriately in response to exercise. The HR vs. $\dot{V}O_2$ curve will generally have a steeper slope (left shift) compared with control; Figure 9.12b. In patients with lung disease, the predicted HR max is usually not reached and their HR reserve is then increased; Figure 9.12c. Patients with chronotropic incompetence (i.e., cannot increase HR appropriately), such as patients with pacemakers, those on β-blockers, or patients with severe

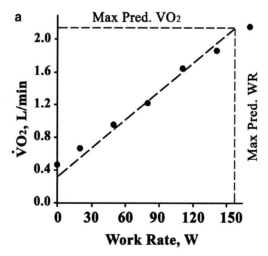

FIGURE 9.11. $\dot{V}O_2$ vs. WR curve; (**a**) Patient achieved predicted max $\dot{V}O_2$; (**b**) Patient did not achieve the predicted max $\dot{V}O_2$, indicating exercise limitation; (**c**) Patient did not achieve the predicted max $\dot{V}O_2$ with an early plateau, indicating reaching $\dot{V}O_2$ max and exercise limitation most likely related to a cardiovascular disease (With permission from ATS/ACCP Statement on Cardiopulmonary Exercise Testing. Am J Respir Crit Care Med 2003;167:211–277.)

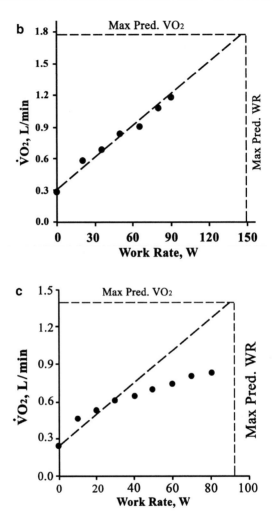

FIGURE 9.11 (continued)

HF,[142,159] may have a high HR reserve but are still limited by their cardiovascular system.

- The O_2 pulse, which is representative of the SV, is generally decreased at peak exercise in patients with heart disease and its curve shows an early plateau; Figure 9.12b. In normal patients and in patients with lung disease, however, the O_2 pulse is usually normal; Figure 9.12a, c.

- The AT is reached earlier than predicted (40–60% of predicted peak $\dot{V}O_2$) in patients with heart disease. In patients with lung disease, however, it is normal, indeterminate, or not reached as the patient may stop prematurely due to ventilatory limitation. AT can be determined from $\dot{V}E$, $\dot{V}CO_2$, $\dot{V}E/\dot{V}O_2$, or $P_{ET}O_2$ curves; Figure 9.4.
- An early plateau of the $\dot{V}O_2$ vs. WR curve (i.e., $\downarrow\Delta\dot{V}O_2/\Delta WR$ ratio) also suggests a cardiovascular limitation to exercise; Figure 9.11c.[160,161]
- An abnormal BP response (excessive rise, failure to rise or drop in BP) suggests a cardiovascular abnormality.
- Exercise-related significant ECG changes (arrhythmia or ischemia) suggest a cardiac disease.

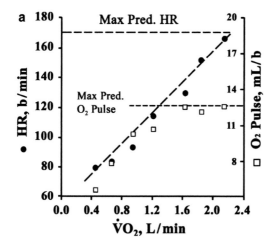

FIGURE 9.12. HR and O_2 pulse vs. $\dot{V}O_2$ curves; (**a**) HR and O_2 pulse curves along the predicted curves, indicating normal response to exercise; (**b**) HR curve shifted to the left with steep slope; O_2 pulse curve has an early plateau indicating a cardiac disease limiting exercise; (**c**) HR and O_2 pulse curves along the predicted curves but with increased HR reserve. This pattern can be seen in submaximal effort and in respiratory disease (With permission from ATS/ACCP Statement on Cardiopulmonary Exercise Testing. Am J Respir Crit Care Med 2003;167:211–277.).

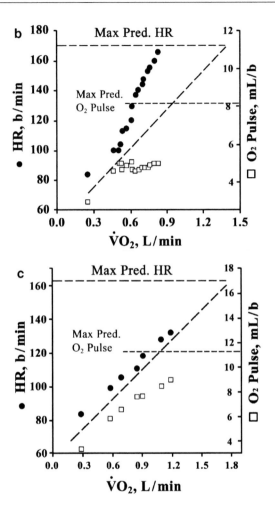

<figure>FIGURE 9.12. (continued)</figure>

Respiratory System

• *Ventilatory response*: Determine whether the ventilatory response is normal by looking at V̇E max, breathing (and/or ventilatory) reserve, RR and tidal FV loops:
  – The measured V̇E max is normally much less than the calculated MVV (the calculated MVV should equal or be close

to the predicted MVV in normal subjects); Figure 9.13a. In ventilatory disease, however, $\dot{V}E$ max approaches or even exceeds the calculated MVV, which is shown as a shift to the left in $\dot{V}E$ curve; Figure 9.13b. The calculated MVV itself is much reduced compared with the predicted MVV in these patients.

- The breathing reserve ($\dot{V}E$ max/calculated MVV) is usually close to 1 in patients with ventilatory disease and is much lower in normal subjects and in patients with a pure cardiac disease. There is normally a significant ventilatory ($\dot{V}E$) reserve (calculated MVV – $\dot{V}E$ max), which is reduced in ventilatory disease.
- RR often increases excessively in ventilatory disease.
- In COPD, evidence of dynamic hyperinflation in the tidal FV loops indicates a ventilatory limitation to exercise; Figure 9.10. This is not seen normally or in patients with isolated heart disease.

• *Gas-exchange response*: Determine whether the gas-exchange response is normal by looking at V_D/V_T, $P_{ET}CO_2$ (and P_aCO_2), S_pO_2, and the ABG at exercise termination (if measured).

- V_D/V_T fails to drop as expected or even increases in patients with a gas-exchange abnormality in response to exercise, while it decreases in normal subjects. It may behave abnormally with exercise in patients with a significant cardiac disease because of impaired lung perfusion.
- A gas-exchange disorder can result in abnormal increase in P_aCO_2 and $P_{ET}CO_2$ at peak exercise, while they normally decrease. Similarly, these variables increase with a ventilatory disease.
- In patients with a gas-exchange abnormality, P_aO_2 is reduced and $P_{(A-a)}O_2$ is increased (>35 mmHg) because of impaired gas exchange and $\dot{V}/Q$ mismatch, while P_aO_2 remains stable normally during exercise. $P_{(A-a)}O_2$ may show a slight increase in normal subjects as a result of $\dot{V}/Q$ mismatching, O_2 diffusion limitation, and low mixed venous O_2.[162]
- Similarly, S_pO_2 (and S_aO_2) is unchanged in most normal subjects during exercise but may drop in gas-exchange disturbances.

• Tables 9.7 and 9.8 show the classic findings in pure cardiac and pulmonary disease in a stepwise approach. Table 9.9 summarizes the exercise patterns of other common conditions.

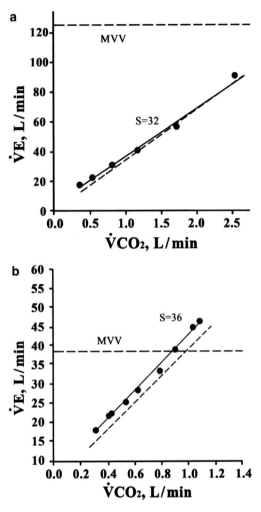

FIGURE 9.13. $\dot{V}E$ vs. $\dot{V}CO_2$ curve (this curve serves the same purpose as $\dot{V}E$ vs. $\dot{V}O_2$ curve); (**a**) a normal patient with normal curve (*solid* curve), along the predicted (*dashed*) curve. The calculated MVV (*dashed horizontal line*) here equals the predicted MMV. Note the significant ventilatory reserve; (**b**) a patient with ventilatory limitation with a left shift of the curve compared with the predicted (*dashed*) curve. The calculated MVV (*dashed horizontal line*) is much lower than the predicted MVV (not shown in this figure), and there is no ventilatory reserve (With permission from ATS/ACCP Statement on Cardiopulmonary Exercise Testing. Am J Respir Crit Care Med 2003;167:211–277.)

TABLE 9.7. Pattern in pure cardiac disease such as cardiomyopathy

The base-line spirometry and maximal flow volume loop are usually normal.
Exercise capacity is reduced:
    ↓ peak $\dot{V}O_2$ (<83% predicted)
    Maximum WR is usually ↓.
    The reason for exercise termination is usually fatigue because of early
        AT, but it could be dyspnea related to left ventricular failure.
The cardiovascular response is abnormal:
    HR response
        HR max is usually achieved early (>90% predicted)
        No HR reserve (<15)
        HR curve is steep (left shifted)
    O_2 pulse at peak $\dot{V}O_2$
        The value of O_2 pulse is decreased (<80% predicted)
        O_2 pulse curve shows an early plateau.
    AT has an early onset (<40% predicted).
    $\dot{V}O_2$ vs. WR curve may show an early plateau.
    The BP may show abnormal response to exercise (abnormally low).
    ECG may show arrhythmia or ischemia.
The ventilatory response is normal (understressed):
    $\dot{V}E$ max is normal (< predicted MVV).
        The calculated MVV usually equals or is close to the predicted MVV.
    $\dot{V}E$ curve is normal (along the predicted curve).
    Ventilatory reserve is normal (>15).
    Breathing reserve is normal or even low because $\dot{V}E$ max is
        decreased (the patient stopped prematurely).
    RR max is normal (<50).
    Tidal FV loops show no evidence of dynamic hyperinflation.
The gas-exchange response is normal:
    Dead space fraction:
        V_D/V_T is reduced with exercise (which is normal) or slightly increased
        because of impaired lung perfusion.
    $P_{ET}CO_2$ (and P_aCO_2) decrease at peak exercise, which is normal.
    RER at peak $\dot{V}O_2$ is normal (1.1–1.3).
    S_pO_2 (and S_aO_2) at peak $\dot{V}O_2$ is normal.
    P_aO_2 and $P_{(A-a)}O_2$ at the end of exercise are usually normal.
Conclusion: reduced exercise capacity with impaired cardiovascular
    response indicating a cardiac origin of exercise limitation.

TABLE 9.8. Pattern in pure pulmonary disease such as COPD and ILD

The base-line spirometry and flow volume loop are generally abnormal.
Exercise capacity is reduced:
    ↓ peak $\dot{V}O_2$ (<83% predicted); reduced WR.
    The reason for exercise termination is usually dyspnea with ↑ Borg scale
        for dyspnea.

(continued)

Table 9.8. (continued)

$\dot{V}E$ max approaching the calculated MVV (mainly with a ventilatory disease).

RER of 1.2 or more (mainly with a gas-exchange disorder).

The cardiovascular response is normal (understressed):

HR response

HR max is not achieved (<90% predicted).

Large HR reserve (>15)

HR curve is normal (along the predicted curve).

O_2 pulse at peak $\dot{V}O_2$

The value of O_2 pulse is normal (>80% predicted).

O_2 pulse curve is normal (along the predicted curve).

AT is normal (>40% predicted) or indeterminate if patient stops before reaching AT because of severe ventilatory limitation.

The BP response is normal.

ECG is usually normal.

The ventilatory response is abnormal (typically in a ventilatory disease as COPD):

$\dot{V}E$ max is high (reaching the calculated MVV).

The calculated MVV is much less than the predicted MVV.

$\dot{V}E$ curve is shifted upward and to the left.

No ventilatory reserve (<15).

Breathing reserve ($\dot{V}E$ max/MVV) is increased, can be >1.

RR max is $\uparrow$ (typically very high in patients with ILD because of $\downarrow V_T$).

In COPD, tidal FV loops may show evidence of dynamic hyperinflation.

The gas-exchange response is abnormal (typically in a gas-exchange disorder as ILD):

Dead space fraction:

V_D/V_T is $\uparrow$ at rest and only drops slightly with exercise. It may even increase.

$\dot{V}E/\dot{V}CO_2$ at AT is increased (>34).

$P_{ET}CO_2$ and P_aCO_2 are increased at peak exercise.

RER at peak $\dot{V}O_2$ may be increased.

S_pO_2 (and S_aO_2) at peak $\dot{V}O_2$ may be reduced ($\geq$5%).

ABG at peak $\dot{V}O_2$ may show $\downarrow P_aO_2$ and $\uparrow\uparrow P_{(A-a)}O_2$ (>35).

Conclusion: reduced exercise capacity with impaired ventilatory, gas exchange, or both responses to exercise indicating a pulmonary origin of exercise limitation.

Illustrative Examples

Case 1

A 37-year-old male, Caucasian, presented with shortness of breath. The history and the physical examination were unremarkable. The initial investigations, including a chest X-ray, ECG, and a detailed

TABLE 9.9. Exercise test pattern in other common conditions

Pulmonary hypertension
Exercise capacity is ↓.
The cardiovascular response is abnormal (similar to pure cardiac disease).
Ventilatory response may be normal (lung parenchyma is normal).
Gas-exchange response is abnormal: ↑ resting V_D/V_T with minor drop or even increase with exercise; $P_{(A-a)}O_2$ increases and P_aO_2 drops with exercise.

Myopathy
Exercise capacity is ↓.
The cardiovascular response is abnormal (similar to pure cardiac disease).
Ventilatory response is abnormal [similar to pure lung disease but without complete ventilatory limitation based on V̇E/MVV (it is <1 here)].
Gas-exchange response is normal.

Obesity
Exercise capacity is ↓ in L/min/kg but normal in l/min. The $\dot{V}O_2$ vs. WR curve is more upright than normal.
The cardiovascular response is normal.
Ventilatory response is normal.
Gas-exchange response is normal.

Deconditioning
Exercise capacity is ↓.
The cardiovascular response is borderline – abnormal (HR max is reached earlier than normal and O_2 pulse is not profoundly reduced and may course along the predicted curve, except that it does not reach its peak because of early exercise termination). AT is reduced.
Ventilatory response is normal.
Gas-exchange response is normal.

Malingering
Exercise capacity is ↓ with no obvious reason.
The cardiovascular response is normal.
Ventilatory response is normal.
Gas-exchange response: normal.

lung function study, were normal. A CPET was performed to determine the cause of the patient's shortness of breath. Weight 70 kg; height 184 cm.
- Test details
  - *Instrument*: Cycle ergometer
  - *Technique*: Incremental
  - *Reason for exercise termination*: leg fatigue.
  - *Modified Borg scale*: for dyspnea (8); for leg discomfort (9)
  - *ECG*: normal throughout exercise.

- *Spirometry*

FVC	5.60 (pred.)	4.84 (measured)	86 (% pred.)
FEV_1	4.52 (pred.)	4.30 (measured)	95 (% pred.)
FEV_1/FVC ratio		89%	
MVV**	158 (pred.)	150 (calculated)	

- *Resting data*

HR	80 bpm
BP	116/76 mmHg
S_pO_2	99%
V_D/V_T	0.24

- *Cardiovascular response at peak exercise*

	Pred.	Measured	% Pred.
O_2/kg (ml/kg/min)	39.6	38.0	96
O_2 (L/min)	3.01	3.05	101
WR (Watts)	254	250	98
HR (BPM)	176	181	102
O_2 pulse (ml/beat)	18.9	19.0	101
AT		1.9	65%[††]
CO_2 (L/min)	3.30	3.20	97
BP (mmHg)		180/90	

- *Ventilatory response at peak exercise*

	Pred.	Measured	% Pred.
$\dot{V}E$ (L/min)	150	92	61
V_T (liters)	2.27	2.19	96
RR (cycle/min)		29	
Tidal FV loops		normal throughout exercise	

- *Gas-exchange response at peak exercise*

	Pred.	Measured	% Pred.
$P_{ET}CO_2$ (mmHg)		35	
V_D/V_T	0.18	0.13	72
$\dot{V}E/\dot{V}O_2$ at AT		27	
$\dot{V}E/\dot{V}CO_2$ at AT		25	
S_pO_2 (%)		99	
RER		1.14	

**The conversion factor used in these cases is 35 (not 40).

[††]As a percentage of $\dot{V}O_2$ max.

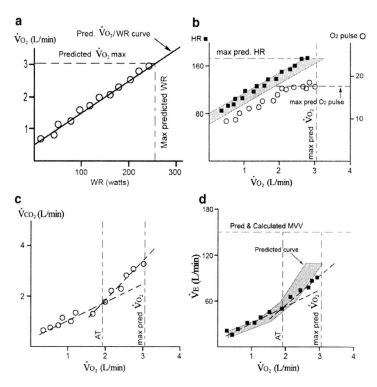

FIGURE 9.14. (a) $\dot{V}O_2$ vs. WR curve; (b) HR and O_2 pulse vs. $\dot{V}O_2$ curves; (c) $\dot{V}CO_2$ vs. $\dot{V}O_2$ curve; (d) $\dot{V}E$ vs. $\dot{V}O_2$ curve.

• For the graphic representation of the patient's data, see Figure 9.14.

Interpretation

• The test was performed because the resting data could not explain the patient's symptoms. The instrument used is a cycle ergometer with an incremental WR. Exercise was terminated because of leg discomfort that scored 9/12 in the modified Borg scale, while dyspnea scored 8/12.

• Base-line spirometry was normal.

- The patient achieved a maximal effort as evident by
  - Achieving predicted $\dot{V}O_2$ max (101% pred.); see also Figure 9.14a.
  - Achieving predicted maximum WR (98% pred.); Figure 9.14a.
  - Achieving predicted maximum HR (102% pred.); see also Figure 9.14b.
  - Patient's exhaustion; scoring 9/12 for leg discomfort in modified Borg scale at peak exercise.
- The exercise capacity was normal as:
  - Peak $\dot{V}O_2$ was >83% of the predicted $\dot{V}O_2$ max. Peak $\dot{V}O_2$ even exceeded the predicted value of $\dot{V}O_2$ max (101%). This fact can also be shown in $\dot{V}O_2$ vs. WR curve, Figure 9.14a, as the peak $\dot{V}O_2$ approached the predicted $\dot{V}O_2$ max.
  - Similarly, the predicted maximum WR had been achieved (98% pred.); Figure 9.14a.
- Cardiovascular response:
  - The HR response was normal as:
    (a) HR max was 102% pred. (the normal is >90% pred.).
    (b) There was no HR reserve (176–181 = –5, which is normal).
    (c) HR curve is along the predicted curve; Figure 9.14b.
  - O_2 pulse at peak exercise was normal (101% pred.) and its curve is along the predicted one; Figure 9.14b.
  - AT as determined from $\dot{V}CO_2$ vs. $\dot{V}O_2$ curve ($\dot{V}$ slope) and $\dot{V}E$ vs. $\dot{V}O_2$ curve, Figure 9.14c, d, was found to be 1.9 L/min (65% of $\dot{V}O_2$ max), which is normal (>40%).
  - $\dot{V}O_2$ vs. WR curve is along the predicted curve; Figure 9.14a.
  - ECG and BP responses were normal.
  - Therefore, the cardiovascular response was normal.
- Ventilatory response:
  - $\dot{V}E$ max was normal (61% pred., which is normally <70% pred.):
    (a) The calculated and predicted MVV are almost identical (150 and 158 L, respectively).
    (b) The $\dot{V}E$ vs. $\dot{V}O_2$ curve is along the predicted one; Figure 9.14d.
    (c) The ventilatory ($\dot{V}E$) reserve was normal (150–90 = 60 which is >15).
    (d) The breathing reserve was also normal (90/150 = 0.6).
  - RR at peak exercise was normal (29).
  - Tidal FV loops were normal with no evidence of dynamic hyperinflation.
  - Therefore, the ventilatory response was normal.

- Gas-exchange response:
  - Dead space fraction at peak exercise was normal:
    (a) V_D/V_T dropped from 0.24 (at rest) to 0.13 (at peak exercise), which is a normal response.
    (b) $\dot{V}E/\dot{V}CO_2$ and $\dot{V}E/\dot{V}O_2$ at AT were normal (25 and 27, respectively).
  - $P_{ET}CO_2$ at peak exercise was normal.
  - RER at peak exercise was 1.14, which is normal.
  - S_pO_2 had remained normal throughout exercise (99%).[‡‡]
  - Therefore, the gas-exchange response was normal.
- Conclusion
    (a) There was no evidence of exercise limitation. The study is normal.

Case 2

A 31-year-old male, Caucasian, a known case of pulmonary hypertension secondary to pulmonary thromboembolism has recently undergone thromboendarterectomy. A CPET was performed to evaluate the results of this intervention. The patient is also known to have significant emphysema secondary to alpha-1-anti-trypsin deficiency. Weight 121 kg; height 190 cm.

- *Test details*
  - *Instrument*: Cycle ergometer
  - *Technique*: Incremental
  - *Reason for exercise termination*: dyspnea.
  - *Modified Borg scale*: for dyspnea (9); for leg discomfort (9)
  - *ECG*: normal throughout exercise.
- *Spirometry*

FVC	6.09 (pred.)	4.29 (measured)	70 (% pred.)
FEV_1	4.92 (pred.)	2.23 (measured)	45 (% pred.)
FEV_1/FVC ratio		52%	
MVV	172 (pred.)	78 (calculated)	

- *Resting data*

HR	95 bpm
BP	117/75 mmHg
S_pO_2	100%
V_D/V_T	0.39

[‡‡] Comment on the ABG result before and after exercise especially P_aO_2, P_aCO_2, and $P_{(A-a)}O_2$ if ABG is available.

- *Cardiovascular response at peak exercise*

	Pred.	Measured	% Pred.
$\dot{V}O_2$/kg (ml/kg/min)	43	15.7	37
$\dot{V}O_2$ (L/min)	4.5	1.9	42
WR (Watts)	287	132	46
HR (BPM)	181	148	82
O_2 pulse (ml/beat)	21.0	12.9	61
AT		1.4	29%[§§]
$\dot{V}CO_2$ (L/min)		2.3	
BP (mmHg)		180/90	

- *Ventilatory response at peak exercise*

	Pred.	Measured	% Pred.
$\dot{V}E$ (L/min)	78	95	121
V_T (liters)	2.2	2.0	90
RR (cycle/min)		47	

- Gas-exchange response at peak exercise

	Pred.	Measured	% Pred.
$P_{ET}CO_2$ (mmHg)		26.4	
V_D/V_T	0.18	0.13	72
$\dot{V}E/\dot{V}O_2$ at AT		36	
$\dot{V}E/\dot{V}CO_2$ at AT		36	
S_pO_2 (%)		95	
RER		1.2	

- For the graphic representation of the patient's data, see Figure 9.15.

[§§]As a percentage of $\dot{V}O_2$ max.

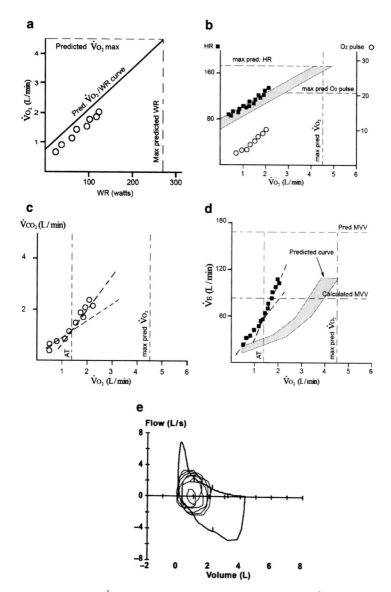

FIGURE 9.15.   (a) $\dot{V}O_2$ vs. WR curve; (b) HR and O_2 pulse vs. $\dot{V}O_2$ curves; (c) $\dot{V}CO_2$ vs. $\dot{V}O_2$ curve; (d) $\dot{V}E$ vs. $\dot{V}O_2$ curve; (e) Tidal FV loops during exercise within the maximal FV loop

Interpretation

- Incremental CPET using a cycle ergometer was performed to assess the response to endarterectomy. Exercise was terminated because of dyspnea that scored 9/12 in the modified Borg scale; leg discomfort similarly scored 9/12.
- Base-line spirometry shows severe obstructive defect indicating that the patient's emphysema is severe.
- The patient achieved a maximal effort as evident by
  - Patient's exhaustion – scoring 9 for dyspnea and leg discomfort in the modified Borg scale.
  - Exceeding the calculated MVV; see Figure 9.15d.
  - Achieving a RER of 1.2.
- The exercise capacity was moderately–severely reduced as follows:
  - Peak $\dot{V}O_2$ was only 42% of the predicted $\dot{V}O_2$ max, and the achieved WR at peak exercise was only 46% of the predicted maximum WR. These features are also noticed in the $\dot{V}O_2$ vs. WR curve; Figure 9.15a.
  - Because the patient is obese (121 kg), it is important to correct $\dot{V}O_2$ for weight by examining $\dot{V}O_2$/kg, which still indicates a marked reduction in exercise capacity (37%).
- Cardiovascular response:
  - The HR response was normal although the patient did not achieve his maximum predicted HR as he needed to terminate exercise prematurely because of ventilatory limitation:
    - (a) HR max was 82% pred., which is abnormally low (normal >90% pred.).
    - (b) Increased HR reserve (181 – 148 = 33).
    - (c) HR curve is along the predicted curve; Figure 9.15b.
  - O_2 pulse at peak exercise was low (61% pred.). The curve is showing an early plateau; Figure 9.15b. The decreased stroke volume response could be due to deconditioning or reduced O_2 carrying capacity.
  - AT was low (1.4 or 29% of predicted $\dot{V}O_2$ max) as determined from $\dot{V}CO_2$ vs. $\dot{V}O_2$ and $\dot{V}E$ vs. $\dot{V}O_2$ curves; Figure 9.15c, d. The early onset of AT could similarly be related to deconditioning or reduced O_2 carrying capacity.
  - $\dot{V}O_2$ vs. WR curve is parallel to the predicted curve but $\dot{V}O_2$ is slightly lower than expected for any given WR; Figure 9.15a. The curve did not reach a plateau.
  - ECG and BP responses were normal.
  - Therefore, cardiovascular response was normal.

- Ventilatory response:
  - $\dot{V}E$ max was abnormally increased (112% pred.; normal <70% pred.):
    (a) The calculated MVV was much lower than the predicted MVV indicating that the patient had a ventilatory abnormality.
    (b) The $\dot{V}E/\dot{V}O_2$ curve is shifted to the left indicating an abnormally increased ventilatory response; Figure 9.15d.
    (c) There was no ventilatory reserve (78–95 = -27; normal >15).
    (d) The breathing reserve was also abnormally high (95/78 = 1.22).
  - RR at peak exercise was increased (47).
  - Tidal FV loops showed dynamic hyperinflation; Figure 9.15e.
  - Therefore, there was an abnormal ventilatory response to exercise.
- Gas-exchange response:
  - Dead space fraction at peak exercise was normal:
    (a) V_D/V_T dropped from 0.39 (at rest) to 0.13 (at peak exercise), which is a normal response.
    (b) $\dot{V}E/\dot{V}CO_2$(31) and $\dot{V}E/\dot{V}O_2$(32) at AT were at the upper limit of normal.
  - $P_{ET}CO_2$ at peak exercise was normal.
  - RER at peak exercise was 1.2, which is normal.
  - S_pO_2 remained normal throughout exercise (99–100%).
  - No ABG was done.
  - Therefore, there was no significant gas-exchange abnormality.
- Conclusion
  - Findings suggest moderate to severe exercise limitation associated with an abnormal ventilatory response, which could be attributed to the significant obstructive disorder (COPD). There was no significant gas-exchange abnormality as dead space fraction behaved normally with exercise as did the S_pO_2. The patient had a normal HR response to exercise but the reduced O_2 pulse and AT suggest deconditioning or reduced O_2 carrying capacity. Lack of an appropriate increase in HR response to compensate for the decreased stroke volume may indicate that the patient was on a β-blocking agent.

Case 3

A 25-year-old female, Caucasian, who is known to have an idiopathic cardiomyopathy, underwent a CPET to assess the need for a cardiac transplant. Weight 68 kg; height 171 cm.

- *Test details*
  - Instrument: Cycle ergometer
  - Technique: Incremental
  - Reason for exercise termination: fatigue.
  - Modified Borg scale: for dyspnea (6); for leg discomfort (9).
  - ECG: normal throughout exercise.
- *Spirometry*

FVC	4.27 (pred.)	3.39 (measured)	80 (% pred.)
FEV_1	3.41 (pred.)	2.93 (measured)	81 (% pred.)
FEV_1/FVC ratio		86%	
MVV	119 (pred.)	103 (Calculated)	

- *Resting data*

HR	94 bpm
BP	123/78 mmHg
S_pO_2	96%
V_D/V_T	0.36

- *Cardiovascular response at peak exercise*

	Pred.	*Measured*	*% Pred.*
$\dot{V}O_2$/kg (ml/kg/min)	39	21	54
$\dot{V}O_2$ (L/min)	3.4	1.4	41
WR (Watts)	170	96	57
HR (BPM)	182	189	104
O_2 pulse (ml/beat)	11.9	7.1	59
AT		0.74	21%
$\dot{V}CO_2$ (L/min)		1.7	
BP (mmHg)		137/88	

- *Ventilatory response at peak exercise*

	Pred.	Measured	% Pred.
$\dot{V}E$ (L/min)	103	65	68
V_T (liters)	1.5	1.9	124
RR (cycle/min)		35	

Gas-exchange response at peak exercise

	Pred.	Measured	% Pred.
$P_{ET}CO_2$ (mmHg)		31.5	
V_D/V_T	0.18	0.13	72
$\dot{V}E/\dot{V}O_2$ at AT		31	
$\dot{V}E/\dot{V}CO_2$ at AT		36	
S_pO_2 (%)		95	
RER		1.2	

- For the graphic representation of the patient's data, see Figure 9.16.

Interpretation

- An incremental CPET using a cycle ergometer was performed to assess the need for a cardiac transplant. Exercise was terminated because of fatigue. The modified Borg score for dyspnea and leg discomfort was 9/12.
- Base-line spirometry was normal.
- The patient achieved a maximal effort as evident by:
  - Patient's exhaustion, scoring 9/12 for both dyspnea and leg discomfort in modified Borg scale at peak exercise.
  - Reaching a plateau in the $\dot{V}O_2$ vs. WR curve; Figure 9.16a.
  - Achieving predicted maximum HR (102%); see also Figure 9.16b.
  - Achieving a RER of 1.2.
- The exercise capacity was moderately to severely reduced as:

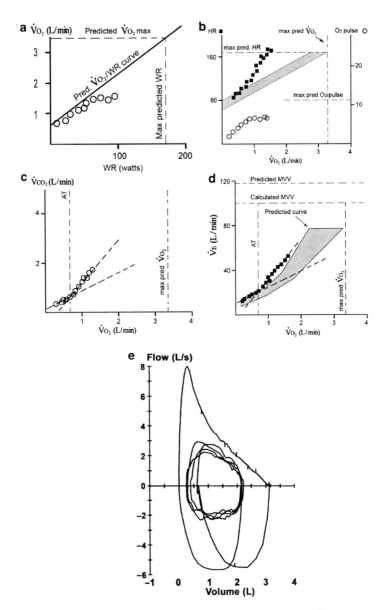

FIGURE 9.16. (a) $\dot{V}O_2$ vs. WR curve; (b) HR and O_2 pulse vs. $\dot{V}O_2$ curves; (c) $\dot{V}CO_2$ vs. $\dot{V}O_2$ curve; (d) $\dot{V}E$ vs. $\dot{V}O_2$ curve; (e) Tidal FV loops during exercise within the maximal FV loop.

(a) Peak $\dot{V}O_2$ was 41% of the predicted $\dot{V}O_2$ max, see also $\dot{V}O_2$ vs. WR curve; Figure 9.16a.

(b) Similarly, the WR achieved was low (57% pred.); see Figure 9.16a.

- Cardiovascular response:
  - The HR response was abnormally increased as:
    (a) The resting HR was increased (94/min).
    (b) The maximum predicted HR was achieved prematurely. HR max was 104% pred. with no HR reserve (189 − 182 = −7).
    (c) HR curve is steep and shifted to the left; Figure 9.16b.
  - O_2 pulse at peak exercise was reduced (59% pred.) and its curve shows an early plateau; Figure 9.16b.
  - AT was achieved prematurely (0.74 L/min, 21% of $\dot{V}O_2$ max); Figure 9.16c, d. An early AT suggests a cardiovascular compromise.
  - $\dot{V}O_2$ vs. WR curve demonstrates an early plateau (i.e. $\downarrow\Delta\dot{V}O_2/\Delta WR$ ratio); Figure 9.16a.
  - BP response to exercise was abnormally low. The ECG was normal throughout exercise.
  - These findings suggest that a cardiac disease is responsible for exercise limitation.
- Ventilatory response:
  - $\dot{V}E$ max was normal (61% pred., which should normally be <70% pred.):
    (a) The calculated and predicted MVV were within the acceptable range of normal (103 and 119 L, respectively).
    (b) The $\dot{V}E$ vs. $\dot{V}O_2$ curve was along the predicted one with a small shift to the left; Figure 9.16d.
    (c) Ventilatory reserve was 103 − 65 = 48, which is high (>15), indicating that exercise was terminated early.
    (d) The breathing reserve was also high (65/103 = 0.63).
  - RR at peak exercise was 35/min.
  - The tidal FV loops were way away from the maximal FV loop suggesting significant ventilatory reserve.
  - The earlier findings suggest that the ventilatory system was understressed and its response to exercise was generally normal.
- Gas-exchange response:
  - Dead space fraction at peak exercise was normal:
    (a) V_D/V_T dropped from 0.36 (at rest) to 0.13 (at peak exercise), which is a normal response.

(b) $\dot{V}E/\dot{V}CO_2$ and $\dot{V}E/\dot{V}O_2$ at AT were elevated (36 and 36, respectively).
- $P_{ET}CO_2$ at peak exercise was normal.
- RER at peak exercise was normal (1.2).
- S_pO_2 remained normal throughout exercise (95%).
- The slightly impaired gas exchange may suggest impaired lung perfusion secondary to cardiomyopathy.
- Conclusion
  - There was moderate to severe exercise limitation associated with an abnormal cardiovascular response. Findings also suggest some degree of gas-exchange abnormality, which may be explained by impaired pulmonary perfusion.

Case 4

A 62-year-old male, Caucasian, with known idiopathic pulmonary fibrosis (IPF) undergoing a CPET as part of lung transplant workup. The patient is on 24-h O_2 therapy at 5 l/min through nasal prongs. Weight 79 kg; height 168 cm.
- *Test details*
  - *Instrument*: Cycle ergometer
  - *Technique*: Incremental
  - *Reason for exercise termination*: dyspnea
  - *Modified Borg scale*: for dyspnea (10); for leg discomfort (5)
  - *ECG*: normal throughout exercise
- *Spirometry*

FVC	4.10 (pred.)	1.97 (measured)	48 (% pred.)
FEV_1	3.25 (pred.)	1.35 (measured)	41 (% pred.)
FEV_1/FVC ratio		68%	
MVV	114 (pred.)	47 (calculated)	

- *Resting data*

HR	92 bpm
BP	120/78 mmHg
S_pO_2	98% (on 45% F_IO_2)
V_D/V_T	0.34

- *Cardiovascular response at peak exercise*

	Pred.	Measured	% Pred.
$\dot{V}O_2$/kg (ml/kg/min)	25.9	15.2	59
$\dot{V}O_2$ (L/min)	2.2	1.2	54
WR (Watts)	151	70	46
HR (BPM)	156	114	73
O_2 pulse (ml/beat)	13.5	11.7	87
AT		Indeterminate	
$\dot{V}CO_2$ (L/min)		1.4	
BP (mmHg)		177/98	

- *Ventilatory response at peak exercise*

	Pred.	Measured	% Pred.
$\dot{V}E$ (L/min)	47	37	79
V_T (liters)	0.68	0.52	74
RR (cycle/min)		48	

- *Gas-exchange response at peak exercise*

	Pred.	Measured	% Pred.
$P_{ET}CO_2$ (mmHg)		44.3	
V_D/V_T	0.18	0.32	135
S_pO_2 (%)		91	
RER		1.29	

- For the graphic representation of the patient's data, see Figure 9.17.

Interpretation

- An incremental CPET using a cycle ergometer was performed as part of lung transplant workup. Exercise was terminated because of dyspnea. The modified Borg score for dyspnea was 10/12 and for leg discomfort was 5/12.
- Base-line spirometry showed severe restriction with a mild obstructive component.

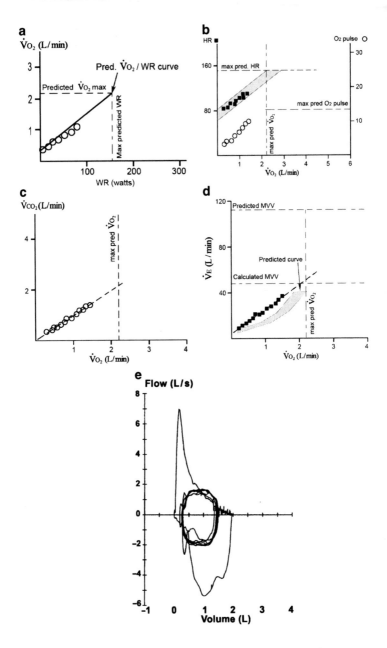

FIGURE 9.17. (a) $\dot{V}_{O_2}$ vs. WR curve; (b) HR and O_2 pulse vs. $\dot{V}_{O_2}$ curves; (c) $\dot{V}_{CO_2}$ vs. $\dot{V}_{O_2}$ curve; (d) $\dot{V}_E$ vs. $\dot{V}_{O_2}$ curve; (e) Tidal FV loops during exercise within the maximal FV loop.

- The patient achieved a maximal effort as evident by:
  - Patient's exhaustion, scoring 10/12 for dyspnea in the modified Borg scale at peak exercise.
  - $\dot{V}E$ max approaching the calculated MVV (>70% of calculated MVV)
  - Achieving a RER of >1.15.
- The exercise capacity was moderately reduced as:
  - Peak $\dot{V}O_2$ was 54% of the predicted $\dot{V}O_2$ max, see also Figure 9.17a.
  - Similarly, the WR achieved was reduced (46% pred.); see Figure 9.17a.
- Cardiovascular response:
  - The HR response was normal:
    (a) Although the resting HR was high (92/min), the maximum predicted HR had not been achieved at peak exercise (73% pred). Therefore, the HR reserve was high (156 − 114 = 42).
    (b) HR curve is running along the predicted curve; Figure 9.17b.
  - O_2 pulse response was normal (87% pred.) and its curve runs along the predicted one; Figure 9.17b.
  - AT could not be determined, which may indicate that it had not been achieved as the cardiovascular system had not been stressed enough before exercise termination; Figure 9.17c, d. This strongly supports a noncardiac cause for exercise limitation.
  - O_2 vs. WR curve was normal; Figure 9.17a.
  - BP and ECG responses to exercise were normal.
  - Therefore, the cardiovascular response to exercise was normal.
- Ventilatory response:
  - $\dot{V}E$ max was high (79% pred., which should normally be <70% pred.):
    (a) The calculated MVV was significantly reduced compared with the predicted one, suggesting a ventilatory disturbance (47 and 114 L, respectively).
    (b) The $\dot{V}E$ vs. $\dot{V}O_2$ curve is slightly shifted to the left; Figure 9.17d.
    (c) Ventilatory reserve was reduced (47 − 37 = 10, which should be >15), while the breathing reserve was normal (37/47 = 0.78).
  - RR at peak exercise was 48/min, which is high. V_T at peak exercise was abnormally reduced.
  - The tidal FV loops were approximating the expiratory envelope of the maximal FV loop but did not show dynamic hyperinflation with shift to the left as is expected with emphysema. This

pattern is compatible with the mechanical disturbance seen in patients with interstitial lung disease.
- Therefore, there was abnormal ventilatory response to exercise as evident by the reduced calculated MVV, reduced ventilatory reserve, and left-shifted $\dot{V}E$ curve. The increased RR with an abnormally reduced VT is in keeping with a restrictive disorder as seen in IPF.
• Gas-exchange response:
  - Dead space fraction at peak exercise was abnormally high:
    ▪ V_D/V_T was high (at rest – 0.34) and remained elevated throughout exercise (0.32) indicating a gas-exchange abnormality.
  - $P_{ET}CO_2$ at peak exercise was high.
  - RER at peak exercise was high (1.29).
  - S_pO_2 has dropped by >5% despite the supplemental O_2 (from 98% to 91%).
  - ABG was not performed.
  - These finding suggest a significant gas-exchange abnormality.
• Conclusion
  - There was moderate exercise limitation associated with an abnormal gas exchange and ventilatory responses to exercise. Both abnormalities likely played a part in the exercise limitation.

References

1. ATS statement: guidelines for the six-minute walk test. ATS Committee on Proficiency Standards for Clinical Pulmonary Function Laboratories. Am J Respir Crit Care Med 2002;166(1):111–117.
2. Solway S, Brooks D, Lacasse Y, Thomas S. A qualitative systematic overview of the measurement properties of functional walk tests used in the cardiorespiratory domain. Chest 2001;119(1):256–270.
3. Solway S, Brooks D, Lacasse Y, Thomas S. A qualitative systematic overview of the measurement properties of functional walk tests used in the cardiorespiratory domain. Chest 2001;119:256–270.
4. Kadikar A, Maurer J, Kesten S. The six-minute walk test: a guide to assessment for lung transplantation. J Heart Lung Transplant 1997;16:313–319.
5. Holden DA, Rice TW, Stelmach K, Meeker DP. Exercise testing, 6 min walk, and stair climb in the evaluation of patients at high risk for pulmonary resection. Chest 1992;102:1774–1779.
6. Sciurba FC, Rogers RM, Keenan RJ, Slivka WA, Gorcsan J III, Ferson PF, Holbert JM, Brown ML, Landreneau RJ. Improvement in pulmonary function and elastic recoil after lung-reduction surgery for diffuse emphysema. N Engl J Med 1996;334:1095–1099.
7. Criner GJ, Cordova FC, Furukawa S, Kuzma AM, Travaline JM, Leyenson V, O'Brien GM. Prospective randomized trial comparing

bilateral lung volume reduction surgery to pulmonary rehabilitation in severe COPD. Am J Respir Crit Care Med 1999;160:2018–2027.

8. Sinclair DJM, Ingram CG. Controlled trial of supervised exercise training in chronic bronchitis. BMJ 1980;280:519–521.

9. Roomi J, Johnson MM, Waters K, Yohannes A, Helm A, Connolly MJ. Respiratory rehabilitation, exercise capacity and quality of life in chronic airways disease in old age. Age Ageing 1996;25:12–16.

10. Paggiaro PL, Dahle R, Bakran I, Frith L, Hollingworth K, Efthimiou J. Multicentre randomised placebo-controlled trial of inhaled fluticasone propionate in patients with COPD. Lancet 1998;351:773–780.

11. Leggett RJ, Flenley DC. Portable oxygen and exercise tolerance in patients with chronic hypoxic cor pulmonale. BMJ 1977;2:84–86.

12. Spence DPS, Hay JG, Carter J, Pearson MG, Calverley PMA. Oxygen desaturation and breathlessness during corridor walking in COPD: effect of oxitropium bromide. Thorax 1993;48:1145–1150.

13. DeBock V, Mets T, Romagnoli M, Derde MP. Captopril treatment of chronic heart failure in the very old. J Gerontol 1994;49:M148–M152.

14. O'Keeffe ST, Lye M, Donnnellan C, Carmichael DN. Reproducibility and responsiveness of quality of life assessment and six minute walk test in elderly heart failure patients. Heart 1998;80:377–382.

15. Bernstein ML, Despars JA, Singh NP, Avalos K, Stansbury DW, Light RW. Re-analysis of the 12 minute walk in patients with COPD. Chest 1994;105:163–167.

16. Hajiro T, Nishimura K, Tsukino M, Ikeda A, Koyama H, Izumi T. Analysis of clinical methods used to evaluate dyspnea in patients with COPD. Am J Respir Crit Care Med 1998;158:1185–1189.

17. Gulmans VAM, vanVeldhoven NHMJ, deMeer K, Helders PJM. The six-minute walking test in children with cystic fibrosis: reliability and validity. Pediatr Pulmonol 1996;22:85–89.

18. Nixon PA, Joswiak ML, Fricker FJ. A six-minute walk test for assessing exercise tolerance in severely ill children. J Pediatr 1996;129:362–366.

19. Bittner V. Six-minute walk test in patients with cardiac dysfunction. Cardiologia 1997;42:897–902.

20. Peeters P, Mets T. The 6 minute walk as an appropriate exercise test in elderly patients with chronic heart failure. J Gerontol 1996;51A:M147–M151.

21. Zugck C, Kruger C, Durr S, Gerber SH, Haunstetter A, Hornig K, Kubler W, Haass M. Is the 6-minute walk test a reliable substitute for peak oxygen uptake in patients with dilated cardiomyopathy? Eur Heart J 2000;21:540–549.

22. Bittner V, Weiner DH, Yusuf S, Rogers WJ, McIntyre KM, Bangdiwala SI, Kronenberg MW, Kostis JB, Kohn RM, Guillotte M, et al. Prediction of mortality and morbidity with a 6-minute walk test in patients with left ventricular dysfunction. JAMA 1993;270:1702–1707.

23. Cahalin LP, Mathier MA, Semigran MJ, Dec GW, DiSalvo TG. The sixminute walk test predicts peak oxygen uptake and survival in patients with advanced heart failure. Chest 1996;110:325–332.

24. Cote CG, Celli BR. In patients with COPD, the 6 minute walking distance is a better predictor of health care utilization than FEV1, blood gases, and dyspnea [abstract]. Eur Respir J 1998;383.
25. Kessler R, Faller M, Fourgaut G, Mennecier B, Weitzenblum E. Predictive factors of hospitalization for acute exacerbation in a series of 64 patients with chronic obstructive pulmonary disease. Am J Respir Crit Care Med 1999;159:158–164.
26. Cahalin L, Pappagianopoulos P, Prevost S, Wain J, Ginns L. The relationship of the 6-min walk test to maximal oxygen consumption in transplant candidates with end-stage lung disease. Chest 1995;108:452–459.
27. Enright PL, McBurnie MA, Bittner V, Tracy RP, McNamara R, Newman AB. the Cardiovascular Health Study. The six minute walk test: a quick measure of functional status in elderly adults. Chest 2003;123:387–398.
28. Enright PL, Sherrill DL. Reference equations for the six-minute walk in healthy adults. Am J Respir Crit Care Med 1998;158:1384–1387.
29. Barst RJ, Rubin LJ, McGoon MD, Caldwell EJ, Long WA, Levy PS. Survival in primary pulmonary hypertension with long-term continuous intravenous prostacyclin. Ann Intern Med 1994;121:409–415.
30. Miyamoto S, Nagaya N, Satoh T, Kyotani S, Sakamaki F, Fujita M, Nakanishi N, Miyatake K. Clinical correlates and prognostic significance of six-minute walk test in patients with primary pulmonary hypertension. Am J Respir Crit Care Med 2000;161:487–492.
31. Guyatt GH, Sullivan MJ, Thompson PJ, Fallen EL, Pugsley SO, Taylor DW, Berman LB. The 6-minute walk: a new measure of exercise capacity in patients with chronic heart failure. Can Med Assoc J 1985;132:919–923.
32. Lipkin DP, Scrivin AJ, Crake T, Poole-Wilson PA. Six minute walking test for assessing exercise capacity in chronic heart failure. BMJ 1986;292:653–655.
33. Troosters T, Gosselink R, Decramer M. Six minute walking distance in healthy elderly subjects. Eur Respir J 1999;14:270–274.
34. Weiss RA, et al. Six minute walk test in severe COPD: reliability and effect of walking course layout and length. Paper presented at ACCP Conference, San Francisco, September 2000.
35. Stevens D, Elpern E, Sharma K, Szidon P, Ankin M, Kesten S. Comparison of hallway and treadmill six-minute walk tests. Am J Respir Crit Care Med 1999;160:1540–1543.
36. Enright PL. The six-minute walk test. Respir Care 2003;48:783–785.
37. Guyatt GH, Pugsley SO, Sullivan MJ, Thompson PJ, Berman LB, Jones NL, Fallen EL, Taylor DW. Effect of encouragement on walking test performance. Thorax 1984;39:818–822.
38. Jensen LA, Onyskiw JE, Prasad NGN. Meta-analysis of arterial oxygen saturation monitoring by pulse oximetry in adults. Heart Lung 1998;27:387–408.
39. Barthelemy JC, Geyssant A, Riffat J, Antoniadis A, Berruyer J, LaCour JR. Accuracy of pulse oximetry during moderate exercise: a comparative study. Scand J Clin Lab Invest 1990;50:533–539.

40. Borg GAV. Psycho-physical bases of perceived exertion. Med Sci Sports Exerc 1982;14:377–381.

41. Hancox B, Whyte K. Pocket Guide to Lung Function Tests, First Edition. McGraw-Hill, Sydney, 2001.

42. Pellegrino R, Viegi G, Brusasco V, et al. Series "ATS/ERS task force: standardisation of lung function testing." Eur Respir J 2005;26:153–161.

43. Weisman IM, Zeballos RJ. Cardiopulmonary exercise testing. Pulm Crit Care Update 1995;11:1–9.

44. Committee on Exercise Testing. ACC/AHA guidelines for exercise testing: a report of the American College of Cardiology/American Heart Association Task Force on Practice Guidelines. J Am Coll Cardiol 1997;30:260–311.

45. Pratter MR, Curley FJ, Dubois J, Irwin RS. Cause and evaluation of chronic dyspnea in a pulmonary disease clinic. Arch Intern Med 1989;149:2277–2282.

46. Martinez FJ, Stanopoulos I, Acero R, Becker FS, Pickering R, Beamis JF. Graded comprehensive cardiopulmonary exercise testing in the evaluation of dyspnea unexplained by routine evaluation. Chest 1994;105:168–174.

47. Weisman IM, Zeballos RJ. Clinical evaluation of unexplained dyspnea. Cardiologia 1996;41:621–634.

48. Sridhar MK, Carter R, Banham SW, Moran F. An evaluation of integrated cardiopulmonary exercise testing in a pulmonary function laboratory. Scott Med J 1995;40:113–116.

49. Gay SE, Weisman IM, Flaherty KE, Martinez FJ. Cardiopulmonary exercise testing in unexplained dyspnea. In: Weisman IM, Zeballos RJ, eds. Clinical Exercise Testing. Karger, Basel, Switzerland, 2002;81–88.

50. Weisman IM, Zeballos RJ. A step approach to the evaluation of unexplained dyspnea: the role of cardiopulmonary exercise testing. Pulm Perspect 1998;15:8–11.

51. Zeballos RJ, Weisman IM, Connery SM, Bradley JP. Standard treadmill (STE) vs. incremental cycle ergometry (IET) in the evaluation of airway hyperreactivity in unexplained dyspnea [abstract]. Am J Respir Crit Care Med 1999;159:A419.

52. Salzman SH. Cardiopulmonary Exercise Testing. The ACCP Pulmonary Board Review, Northbrook, IL, 2003:363–380.

53. Punzal PA, Ries AL, Kaplan RM, Prewitt LM. Maximum intensity exercise training in patients with chronic obstructive pulmonary disease. Chest 1991;100:618–623.

54. Ries AL. The importance of exercise in pulmonary rehabilitation. Clin Chest Med 1994;15:327–337.

55. Casaburi R, Patessio A, Ioli F, Zanaboni S, Donner CF, Wasserman K. Reductions in exercise lactic acidosis and ventilation as a result of exercise training in patients with obstructive lung disease. Am Rev Respir Dis 1991;143:9–18.

56. Bolliger CT, Jordan P, Soler M, Stulz P, Gradel E, Skarvan K, Elsasser S, Gonon M, Wyser C, Tamm M, et al. Exercise capacity as a predictor of postoperative complications in lung resection candidates. Am J Respir Crit Care Med 1995;151:1472–1480.

57. Bolliger CT, Perruchoud AP. Functional evaluation of the lung resection candidate. Eur Respir J 1998;11:198–212.

58. Morice RC, Peters EJ, Ryan MB, Putnam JB, Ali MK, Roth JA. Redefining the lowest exercise peak oxygen consumption acceptable for lung resection of high risk patients. Chest 1996;110:161S.

59. Howard DK, Iademarco EJ, Trulock EP. The role of cardiopulmonary exercise testing in lung and heart–lung transplantation. Clin Chest Med 1994;15:405–420.

60. Williams RJ, Slater WR. Role of cardiopulmonary exercise in lung and heart–lung transplantation. In: Weisman IM, Zeballos RJ, eds. Progress in Respiratory Research, Vol. 32: Clinical Exercise Testing. Karger, Basel, Switzerland, 2002;254–263.

61. Stelken AM, Younis LT, Jennison SH, Miller DD, Miller LW, Shaw LJ, Kargl D, Chaitman BR. Prognostic value of cardiopulmonary exercise testing using percent achieved of predicted peak oxygen uptake for patients with ischemic and dilated cardiomyopathy. J Am Coll Cardiol 1996;27:345–352.

62. Mancini DM, Eisen H, Kussmaul W, Mull R, Edmunds LH Jr, Wilson JR. Value of peak exercise oxygen consumption for optimal timing of cardiac transplantation in ambulatory patients with heart failure. Circulation 1991;83:778–786.

63. Gallagher CG. Exercise and chronic obstructive pulmonary disease. Med Clin North Am 1990;74:619–641.

64. Gallagher CG. Exercise limitation and clinical exercise testing in chronic obstructive pulmonary disease. Clin Chest Med 1994;15:305–326.

65. Oelberg DA, Kacmarek RM, Pappagianopoulos PP, Ginns LC, Systrom DM. Ventilatory and cardiovascular responses to inspired He–O2 during exercise in chronic obstructive pulmonary disease [see comments]. Am J Respir Crit Care Med 1998;158:1876–1882.

66. Richardson RS, Sheldon J, Poole DC, Hopkins SR, Ries AL, Wagner PD. Evidence of skeletal muscle metabolic reserve during whole body exercise in patients with chronic obstructive pulmonary disease. Am J Respir Crit Care Med 1999;159:881–885.

67. O'Donnell DE, Webb KA. Exertional breathlessness in patients with chronic airflow limitation: the role of lung hyperinflation. Am Rev Respir Dis 1993;148:1351–1357.

68. O'Donnell DE, Magnussen B, Aguilaniu B, Gerken F, Hamilton A, Fluge T. Spiriva (Tiotropium) improves exercise tolerance in COPD. Am J Respir Crit Care Med 2002;165:A227.

69. Janicki JS, Weber KT, Likoff MJ, Fishman AP. Exercise testing to evaluate patients with pulmonary vascular disease. Am Rev Respir Dis 1984;129:S93–S95.

70. D'Alonzo GE, Gianotti L, Dantzker DR. Noninvasive assessment of hemodynamic improvement during chronic vasodilator therapy in obliterative pulmonary hypertension. Am Rev Respir Dis 1986;133:380–384.

71. Systrom DM, Cockrill BA, Hales CA. Exercise testing in patients with pulmonary vascular disease. In: Weisman IM, Zeballos RJ, eds. Clinical Exercise Testing. Karger, Basel, Switzerland, 2002;200–204.

72. Sun XG, Hansen JR, Oudiz RJ, Wasserman K. Exercise pathophysiology in patients with primary pulmonary typertension. Circulation 2001;104:429–435.

73. Agusti C, Xaubet A, Agusti AG, Roca J, Ramirez J, Rodriguez-Roisin R. Clinical and functional assessment of patients with idiopathic pulmonary fibrosis: results of a 3 year follow-up. Eur Respir J 1994;7: 643–650.

74. Xaubet A, Agusti C, Luburich P, Roca J, Monton C, Ayuso MC, Barbera JA, Rodriguez-Roisin R. Pulmonary function tests and CT scan in the management of idiopathic pulmonary fibrosis. Am J Respir Crit Care Med 1998;158:431–436.

75. Nixon PA, Orenstein DM, Kelsey SF, Doershuk CF. The prognostic value of exercise testing in patients with cystic fibrosis. N Engl J Med 1992;327:1785–1788.

76. Moser C, Tirakitsoontorn P, Nussbaum E, Newcomb R, Cooper DM. Muscle size and cardiorespiratory response to exercise in cystic fibrosis. Am J Respir Crit Care Med 2000;162:1823–1827.

77. Cotes JE, Zejda J, King B. Lung function impairment as a guide to exercise limitation in work-related lung disorders. Am Rev Respir Dis 1988;137:1089–1093.

78. Becklake MR, Rodarte JR, Kalica AR. NHLBI workshop summary: scientific issues in the assessment of respiratory impairment. Am Rev Respir Dis 1988;137:1505–1510.

79. Cotes JE. Rating respiratory disability: a report on behalf of a working group of the European Society for Clinical Respiratory Physiology [see comments]. Eur Respir J 1990;3:1074–1077.

80. Cotes JE. Lung Function: Assessment and Application in Medicine, Fifth Edition. Blackwell Scientific, Oxford, 1993;54–58.

81. Smith DD. Pulmonary impairment/disability evaluation: controversies and criticisms. Clin Pulm Med 1995;2:334–343.

82. Sue DY. Exercise testing in the evaluation of impairment and disability. Clin Chest Med 1994;15:369–387.

83. American Thoracic Society. Guidelines for methacholine and exercise challenge testing—1999: official statement of the American Thoracic Society. Am J Respir Crit Care Med 2000;161:309–329.

84. Sterk PJ, Fabbri LM, Quanjer PH, Cockcroft DW, O'Byrne PM, Anderson SD, Juniper EF, Malo JL. Airway responsiveness: standardized challenge testing with pharmacological, physical and sensitizing stimuli in adults. Report of Working Party Standardization of Lung Function Tests, European Community for Steel and Coal. Official statement of the European Respiratory Society. Eur Respir J Suppl 1993;16:53–83.

85. European Respiratory Society. Clinical exercise testing with reference to lung diseases: indications, standardization and interpretation strategies. ERS Task Force on Standardization of Clinical Exercise Testing. Eur Respir J 1997;10:2662–2689.

86. Roca J, Whipp BJ, eds. European Respiratory Society Monograph 6: Clinical Exercise Testing. European Respiratory Society, Lausanne, Switzerland, 1997;164.

87. Garfinkel SK, Kesten S, Chapman KR, Rebuck AS. Physiologic and nonphysiologic determinants of aerobic fitness in mild to moderate asthma. Am Rev Respir Dis 1992;145:741–745.

88. Weisman IM, Zeballos RJ. An integrated approach to the interpretation of cardiopulmonary exercise testing. Clin Chest Med 1994;15:421–445.

89. Wasserman K, Hansen JE, Sue DY, Whipp BJ, Casaburi R. Principles of Exercise Testing and Interpretation: Including Pathophysiology and Clinical Applications, Third Edition. Lippincott Williams & Wilkins, Philadelphia, 1999; xv.

90. Weisman IM, Zeballos RJ. Clinical exercise testing. Clin Chest Med 2001;22:679–701.

91. Jones NL. Clinical Exercise Testing, Third Edition. W. B. Saunders, Philadelphia, 1988; x.

92. Carlin BW, Clausen JL, Ries AL. The effects of exercise testing on the prescription of oxygen therapy. Chest 1994;106:361–365.

93. Dean NC, Brown JK, Himelman RB, Doherty JJ, Gold WM, Stulbarg MS. Oxygen may improve dyspnea and endurance in patients with chronic obstructive pulmonary disease and only mild hypoxemia. Am Rev Respir Dis 1992;146:941–945.

94. American Association for Respiratory Care. AARC clinical practice guideline: exercise testing for evaluation of hypoxemia and/or desaturation. Respir Care 1992;37:907–912.

95. American College of Sports Medicine. ACSM's Guidelines for Exercise Testing and Prescription, Fifth Edition. Williams & Wilkins, Baltimore, MD, 1995; xvi.

96. Mogue LR, Rantala B. Capnometers. J Clin Monit 1988;4:115–121.

97. Clark JS, Votteri B, Ariagno RL, Cheung P, Eichhorn JH, Fallat RJ, Lee SE, Newth CJ, Rotman H, Sue DY. Noninvasive assessment of blood gases. Am Rev Respir Dis 1992;145:220–232.

98. Council on Scientific Affairs, American Medical Association. The use of pulse oximetry during conscious sedation. JAMA 1993;270:1463–1468.

99. Tobin MJ. Respiratory monitoring. JAMA 1990;264:244–251.

100. Zeballos RJ, Weisman IM. Behind the scenes of cardiopulmonary exercise testing. Clin Chest Med 1994;15:193–213.

101. Borg GA. Psychophysical bases of perceived exertion. Med Sci Sports Exerc 1982;14:377–381.

102. Killian KJ, Leblanc P, Martin DH, Summers E, Jones NL, Campbell EJ. Exercise capacity and ventilatory, circulatory, and symptom limitation in patients with chronic airflow limitation. Am Rev Respir Dis 1992;146:935–940.

103. Hamilton AL, Killian KJ, Summers E, Jones NL. Muscle strength, symptom intensity, and exercise capacity in patients with cardiorespiratory disorders. Am J Respir Crit Care Med 1995;152:2021–2031.

104. Jones NL, Killian KJ. Exercise limitation in health and disease. N Engl J Med 2000;343:632–641.

105. Fletcher GF, Froelicher VF, Hartley LH, Haskell WL, Pollock ML. Exercise standards: a statement for health professionals from the American Heart Association. Circulation 1990;82:2286–2322.

106. Hellerstein HK. Specifications for exercise testing equipment. American Heart Association Subcommittee on Rehabilitation Target Activity Group. Circulation 1979;59:849A–854A.

107. Hansen JE, Sue DY, Wasserman K. Predicted values for clinical exercise testing. Am Rev Respir Dis 1984;129:S49–S55.

108. Robinson TE, Sue DY, Huszczuk A, Weiler-Ravell D, Hansen JE. Intra-arterial and cuff blood pressure responses during incremental cycle ergometry. Med Sci Sports Exerc 1988;20:142–149.

109. Bradley P. A model for gas-exchange simulation. J Cardiovasc Pulm Tech 1983;11:33–39.

110. Huszczuk A, Whipp BJ, Wasserman K. A respiratory gas exchange simulator for routine calibration in metabolic studies. Eur Respir 1990;3:465–468.

111. Gore CJ, Catcheside PG, French SN, Bennett JM, Laforgia J. Automated $\dot{V}O2$ max calibrator for open-circuit indirect calorimetry systems. Med Sci Sports Exerc 1997;29:1095–1103.

112. Clark JH, Greenleaf JE. Electronic bicycle ergometer: a simple calibration procedure. J Appl Physiol 1971;30:440–442.

113. Van Praagh E, Bedu M, Roddier P, Coudert J. A simple calibration method for mechanically braked cycle ergometers. Int J Sports Med 1992;13:27–30.

114. Russell JC, Dale JD. Dynamic torquemeter calibration of bicycle ergometers. J Appl Physiol 1986;61:1217–1220.

115. Revill SM, Morgan MD. Biological quality control for exercise testing. Thorax 2000;55:63–66.

116. American College of Sports Medicine. ACSM's Guidelines for Exercise Testing and Prescription, Sixth Edition. Williams & Wilkins, Baltimore, MD, 2000;xvi.

117. Jones NL. Clinical Exercise Testing, Fourth Edition. W. B. Saunders, Philadelphia, 1997;xi.

118. Lollgen H, Ulmer H-V, Crean P, Eds. Recommendations and standard guidelines for exercise testing. Report of the Task Force Conference on Ergometry, Titisee 1987. Eur Heart J 1988;9 Suppl K:1–37.

119. Shepard RJ. Tests of maximum oxygen intake: a critical review. Sports Med 1984;1:99–124.

120. Andersen KL, Shepard RJ, Denolin H, Varnauskas E, Masironi R. Fundamentals of exercise testing. World Health Organization, Geneva, Switzerland, 1971;138.

121. Astrand P-O, Rodahl K. Textbook of Work Physiology: Physiological Bases of Exercise, Third Edition. McGraw Hill, New York, 1986;xii.

122. West JB. Respiratory Physiology, The Essentials. Seventh Edition. Lippincott Williams & Wilkins, Philadelphia, PA, 2005.

123. Rosen MJ. Hypoxemic respiratory failure. The ACCP Pulmonary Board Review, Northbrook, IL, 2005:268–272.

124. Weber KT, Wilson JR, Janicki JS, Likoff MJ. Exercise testing in the evaluation of the patient with chronic cardiac failure. Am Rev Respir Dis 1984;129:S60–S62.

125. Dempsey JA, Babcock MA. An integrative view of limitations to muscular performance. Adv Exp Med Biol 1995;384:393–399.

126. Saltin B. Hemodynamic adaptations to exercise. Am J Cardiol 1985;55:42D–47D.

127. Janicki JS, Sheriff DD, Robotham JL, Wise RA. Cardiac output during exercise: contributions of the cardiac, circulatory and respiratory systems. In: Rowell LB, Shepard JT, eds. Handbook of Physiology, Section 12: Exercise: Regulation and Integration of Multiple Systems. Oxford University Press, New York, 1996;649–704.

128. Lange-Andersen K, Shepard RJ, Denolin H, Varnauskas E, Masironi R. Fundamentals of Exercise Testing. World Health Organization, Geneva, Switzerland, 1971.

129. Weber KT, Wilson JR, Janicki JS, Likoff MJ. Exercise testing in the evaluation of the patient with chronic cardiac failure. Am Rev Respir Dis 1984;129:S60–S62.

130. Johnson BD, Saupe KW, Dempsey JA. Mechanical constraints on exercise hyperpnea in endurance athletes. J Appl Physiol 1992;73:874–886.

131. Johnson BD, Beck KC. Respiratory system responses to dynamic exercise. In: Weiler JM, editor. Allergic and Respiratory Disease in Sports Medicine. Marcel Dekker, New York, 1997;1–34.

132. Dempsey JA, Adams L, Ainsworth DM, Fregosi RF, Gallagher CG, Guz A, Johnson BD, Powers SK. Airway, lung and respiratory muscle function during exercise. In: Rowell LB, Shepard JT, editors. Handbook of Physiology, Section 12: Exercise: Regulation and Integration of Multiple Systems. Oxford University Press, New York, 1996;448–514.

133. Patessio A, Casaburi R, Carone M, Appendini L, Donner CF, Wasserman K. Comparison of gas exchange, lactate, and lactic acidosis thresholds in patients with chronic obstructive pulmonary disease. Am Rev Respir Dis 1993;148:622–626.

134. Beaver WL, Wasserman K, Whipp BJ. Bicarbonate buffering of lactic acid generated during exercise. J Appl Physiol 1986;60:472–478.

135. Hughson RL, Weisiger KH, Swanson GD. Blood lactate concentration increases as a continuous function in progressive exercise. J Appl Physiol 1987;62:1975–1981.

136. Bishop D, Jenkins DG, Mackinnon LT. The relationship between plasma lactate parameters, Wpeak and 1-h cycling performance in women. Med Sci Sports Exerc 1998;30:1270–1275.

137. Casaburi R, Porszasz J, Burns MR, Carithers ER, Chang RS, Cooper CB. Physiologic benefits of exercise training in rehabilitation of patients with severe chronic obstructive pulmonary disease. Am J Respir Crit Care Med 1997;155:1541–1551.

138. Belman MJ, Epstein LJ, Doornbos D, Elashoff JD, Koerner SK, Mohsenifar Z. Noninvasive determinations of the anaerobic threshold: reliability and validity in patients with COPD. Chest 1992;102:1028–1034.

139. Maltais F, LeBlanc P, Jobin J, Berube C, Bruneau J, Carrier L, Breton MJ, Falardeau G, Belleau R. Intensity of training and physiologic adapta-

tion in patients with chronic obstructive pulmonary disease. Am J Respir Crit Care Med 1997;155:555–561.

140. Perloff D, Grim C, Flack J, Frohlich ED, Hill M, McDonald M, Morgenstern B. Human blood pressure determination by sphygmomanometry. Circulation 1993;88:2460–2470.

141. Franciosa JA, Park M, Levine TB. Lack of correlation between exercise capacity and indexes of resting left ventricular performance in heart failure. Am J Cardiol 1981;47:33–39.

142. Weber KT, Janicki JS. Cardiopulmonary exercise testing: physiologic principles and clinical applications. W. B. Saunders, Philadelphia, 1986;xvi.

143. Szlachcic J, Massie BM, Kramer BL, Topic N, Tubau J. Correlates and prognostic implication of exercise capacity in chronic congestive heart failure. Am J Cardiol 1985;55:1037–1042.

144. Dillard TA, Piantadosi S, Rajagopal KR. Prediction of ventilation at maximal exercise in chronic air-flow obstruction. Am Rev Respir Dis 1985;132:230–235.

145. Dillard TA, Hnatiuk OW, McCumber TR. Maximum voluntary ventilation: spirometric determinants in chronic obstructive pulmonary disease patients and normal subjects. Am Rev Respir Dis 1993;147: 870–875.

146. Gallagher CG, Brown E, Younes M. Breathing pattern during maximal exercise and during submaximal exercise with hypercapnia. J Appl Physiol 1987;63:238–244.

147. Hey EN, Lloyd BB, Cunningham DJ, Jukes MG, Bolton DP. Effects of various respiratory stimuli on the depth and frequency of breathing in man. Respir Physiol 1966;1:193–205.

148. American Thoracic Society. Standards for the diagnosis and care of patients with chronic obstructive pulmonary disease. Am J Respir Crit Care Med 1995;152:S77–S121.

149. Johnson BD, Weisman IM, Zeballos RJ, Beck KC. Emerging concepts in the evaluation of ventilatory limitation during exercise: the exercise tidal flow–volume loop. Chest 1999;116:488–503.

150. Johnson BD, Beck KC, Zeballos RJ,Weisman IM. Advances in pulmonary laboratory testing. Chest 1999;116:1377–1387.

151. DeLorey DS, Babb TG. Progressive mechanical ventilatory constraints with aging. Am J Respir Crit Care Med 1999;160:169–177.

152. Bouhuys A. Respiratory dead space. In: Fenn WO, Rahn H, eds. Handbook of Physiology, Section III, Vol. 1: Respiration. American Physiological Society, Washington, DC, 1964;699–714.

153. Bohr C. Ueber die lungenathmung. Skand Arch Physiol 1891;2: 236–268.

154. Johnson BD, Dempsey JA. Demand vs. capacity in the aging pulmonary system. Exerc Sport Sci Rev 1991;19:171–210.

155. Dempsey JA. J.B. Wolffe memorial lecture: is the lung built for exercise? Med Sci Sports Exerc 1986;18:143–155.

156. Ries AL, Farrow JT, Clausen JL. Accuracy of two ear oximeters at rest and during exercise in pulmonary patients. Am Rev Respir Dis 1985;132:685–689.

157. Severinghaus JW, Naifeh KH, Koh SO. Errors in 14 pulse oximeters during profound hypoxia. J Clin Monit 1989;5:72–81.

158. American Thoracic Society. Pulmonary Function Laboratory Management and Procedure Manual. American Thoracic Society, New York, 1998.

159. Francis GS, Goldsmith SR, Ziesche S, Nakajima H, Cohn JN. Relative attenuation of sympathetic drive during exercise in patients with congestive heart failure. J Am Coll Cardiol 1985;5:832–839.

160. Hansen JE, Casaburi R, Cooper DM, Wasserman K. Oxygen uptake as related to work rate increment during cycle ergometer exercise. Eur J Appl Physiol 1988;57:140–145.

161. Jones S, Elliott PM, Sharma S, McKenna WJ, Whipp BJ. Cardiopulmonary responses to exercise in patients with hypertrophic cardiomyopathy. Heart 1998;80:60–67.

162. West JB. Ventilation/Blood Flow and Gas Exchange, Fifth Edition. Blackwell Scientific, Oxford (distributed by Year Book, Chicago, IL), 1990;viii, 120.

163. Beaver WL, Wasserman K, Whipp BJ. A new method for detecting anaerobic threshold by gas exchange. J Appl Physiol 1986;60: 2020–2027.

Chapter 10
Diagnostic Tests for Sleep Disorders

SLEEP-RELATED DISORDERS

The International Classification of Sleep Disorders classifies 84 distinct sleep disorders into four major categories.[1]

1. *Dyssomnias* are characterized by insomnia and excessive daytime sleepiness (hypersomnolence). The respiratory sleep disorders belong to this group.
2. *Parasomnias* are characterized by abnormal behavioral events occurring during sleep such as sleepwalking. Parasomnias typically do not cause insomnia or excessive sleepiness.
3. *Medical-psychiatric sleep disorders* are directly caused by medical, neurologic, or psychiatric (mental) disorders.
4. *Proposed sleep disorders* are sleep disorders that so far have no known key features to distinguish them from normal variants or other sleep disorders.

Respiratory Sleep Disorders (Sleep-Disordered Breathing)

Represent a group of sleep disorders caused by abnormal breathing patterns during sleep and may result in sleep fragmentation and excessive daytime sleepiness. There are two major respiratory sleep disorders:

1. Obstructive sleep apnea/hypopnea (OSA or OSAH)
   - The most prevalent respiratory sleep disorder.[2] OSA affects ~9% of men and ~4% of women.[3] It is characterized by repeated upper airway obstruction during sleep due to a

A. Altalag et al., *Pulmonary Function Tests in Clinical Practice*,
DOI: 10.1007/978-1-84882-231-3_10, © Springer-Verlag London Limited 2009

collapsible upper airway resulting in recurrent arousals and often daytime hypersomnolence. Several risk factors for OSA are identified, obesity being the most important.

- OSA is a significant cause of morbidity and mortality.[4] OSA is associated with cardiovascular disease (hypertension,[5-10] coronary artery disease,[11-16] and arrhythmias[17-22]), cerebrovascular disease,[12-16, 23] diabetes mellitus,[24] lipid abnormalities,[25] and pulmonary vascular disease.[26-29] In addition, the excessive sleepiness caused by OSA is a potential cause of road traffic collisions and industrial accidents, which add to the morbidity and mortality of untreated OSA.[30-32]
- The gold standard in the diagnosis of OSA is polysomnography (sleep study) but other tests may aid in making this diagnosis, as will be discussed later. The treatment of choice for OSA is continuous positive airway pressure (CPAP) applied through the nose and/or mouth during sleep. Other modes of therapy include oral appliances, weight reduction, and surgery (especially if there is an obvious cause for airway obstruction such as enlarged tonsils). Tracheostomy to bypass the upper airway is effective but is generally considered a last resort.
- This chapter will mainly deal with tests used to diagnose OSA.

2. Central sleep apnea syndrome (CSA)
   - Is classified into the following:
     - *CSA with decreased respiratory drive* as in *sleep alveolar hypoventilation syndrome* and neuromuscular disorders.
     - *CSA with periodic breathing pattern* as in *Cheyne-Stokes respiration* (seen mainly with heart failure[33, 34]), hypoxia of high altitude, and in diffuse neurological disorders. This form of CSA is more common and is characterized by a hyperpneic phase of breathing (because of abnormally increased respiratory drive) followed by an apneic phase (due to respiratory alkalosis), repetitive in cycling. As in OSA, arousals are common in CSA but they take place during the hyperpneic phase rather than during the apneic phase. Excessive sleepiness may be a consequence of the arousals.[35]

Conditions That May Mimic Respiratory Sleep Disorders

- Patients with other conditions may present to the respiratory sleep disorders' clinic and may even be misdiagnosed with OSA. Excessive sleepiness is a feature that these conditions share with OSA as do all dyssomnias. These conditions may include narcolepsy, excessive use of sedatives, reduced sleep duration, the upper airway resistant syndrome, depression, and anxiety. Periodic limb movement disorder (PLMD) is another condition that should be considered. The distinction of these disorders is usually made on clinical grounds but specific testing may be necessary; Table 10.1.

TABLE 10.1. Conditions that may mimic respiratory sleep disorders

Narcolepsy
Incidence: 1/2,000[36, 37]; equal prevalence in men and women[38]; Starts at young age, worsens over few years and then persists for life.[39] May coexist with OSA.
Etiology: loss of orexin A and B, neurotransmitters responsible for promotion of wakefulness.
Major clinical features
  Daytime sleepiness: could be so severe that patient may doze off with little warning *"sleep attacks."*
  Hypnagogic hallucinations: are vivid, often frightening hallucinations that occur just as the patient is falling asleep or waking up.
  Sleep paralysis: is a complete inability to move for 1–2 min immediately after awakening. It is usually associated with hypnagogic hallucinations or a feeling of suffocation.
  Cataplexy: is unilateral or bilateral loss of muscle tone triggered usually by some form of excitement and leads to partial or complete collapse.
Diagnosis: clinical and with multiple sleep latency test (MSLT); treated with stimulants.

Periodic limb movement disorder (PLMD)
Repetitive leg jerks (mostly dorsiflexion of the feet) usually accompanied by arousals, sleep fragmentation, and excessive sleepiness. PLMD is sometimes called nocturnal or sleep-related myoclonus, which is a misnomer. More common in older age, incidence is unknown and can be caused by medications such as antidepressants (e.g., venlafaxine)
Diagnosis: clinical and polysomnography (PSG). Treatment: similar to restless leg syndrome (RLS).

Restless leg syndrome (RLS)
An unpleasant deep, creeping or crawling sensation in the legs while patient is sitting or lying with an irresistible urge to move the legs. RLS commonly causes insomnia. The prevalence of moderate–severe form is 2.7%, male:female ratio is 1:2. Most patients with RLS also have PLMD.
Etiology: Primary (idiopathic) and secondary (e.g., secondary to: iron deficiency anemia, end-stage renal disease, diabetes mellitus, Parkinson's disease, pregnancy, connective tissue disease, venous insufficiency).[40-71]

(continued)

TABLE 10.1. (continued)

Diagnosis: clinical, PSG may be helpful. Treatment: correct the cause if any (e.g., treat iron deficiency anemia), benzodiazepines, dopaminergic agents, and opioids (in resistant cases).[72]

Upper airway resistance syndrome (UARS)[73, 74]
Is caused by abnormal narrowing of the upper airways that results in increased resistance to airflow during sleep leading to the "respiratory effort related arousals." UARS is commonly seen in women with certain craniofacial abnormalities. Snoring and excessive daytime sleepiness (due to recurrent arousals) are common features.
Diagnosis may be missed in the PSG unless attention is paid to an unexplained increase in arousal index. When considered, PSG is diagnostic but detecting high esophageal pressures prior to arousals using the esophageal balloon catheter system is pathognomonic. Treatment is continuous positive airway pressure (CPAP) similar to OSA.

Primary (habitual or continuous) snoring without sleep apnea
Patients are typically asymptomatic and present due to complaints from their bed partners. Primary snoring is very common and PSG may be needed to exclude OSA.

Miscellaneous conditions
GI disorders: gastroesophageal reflux disease (GERD), swallowing disorders
Respiratory disorders: nocturnal asthma, COPD, pulmonary fibrosis
Psychiatric disorders: panic attacks, anxiety, depression
Neurological disorders: nocturnal seizures
Others: Drugs (hypnotics), excessive alcohol intake, lack of adequate sleep

POLYSOMNOGRAPHY

Introduction

- Polysomnography (PSG) is a comprehensive diagnostic procedure that allows simultaneous recording of a number of physiologic variables during sleep. A minimum of 12 variables are acquired, which include the following:
  - Central and occipital electroencephalography (EEG)
  - Right and left electrooculography (EOG)
  - Chin electromyography (Chin EMG)
  - Right and left leg EMG
  - Electrocardiography (ECG)
  - Airflow
  - Chest movement and abdominal movement channels
  - Pulse oximetry (S_pO_2)

- Each of these variables is displayed on channels (computer display) and evaluated in a process called *scoring* of the PSG. Scoring converts the data into a meaningful summary that can be readily interpreted. Each group of these variables is used to evaluate different aspects of the PSG:
  1. Sleep stages, arousals, and wakefulness are scored using EEG, EOG, and chin EMG channels.
  2. Respiratory events (apneas or hypopneas) are scored using airflow, chest and abdominal movements, and S_pO_2 channels.
  3. Periodic limb movements (PLMs) are scored using the leg EMG channel.
  4. Miscellaneous channels include ECG, sleep position, and snoring.

SLEEP STAGES, AROUSALS, AND WAKEFULNESS

To discuss the scoring of these variables, it is essential to know the sleep stages. Sleep is classified into the following:

- Rapid eye movement (*REM*) sleep
- *Nonrapid eye movement* (*NREM*) sleep, which is subclassified into the following:
  - *Light sleep* (stages 1 and 2)
  - *Deep sleep* (or slow wave sleep) (stages 3 and 4)
- *Relaxed wakefulness* is the stage that immediately precedes sleep and is referred to as stage wake (W), which is subdivided into the following:
  - Stage W with eyes open
  - Stage W with eyes closed

An arousal is a brief awakening that should meet certain criteria, as will be discussed. The variables used to score sleep stages, arousals, and wakefulness, namely, EEG, EOG, and chin EMG are discussed separately in this section. The information in this section was acquired mainly from the standard manual.[75]

Electroencephalography

Used to record the brain electrical signals, which vary according to the sleep stage.

EEG Electrodes (Leads)

- Six EEG electrodes are placed over the patient's head, three on each side.[*] These electrodes are central, occipital, and auricular

---

[*]The standard EEG recording for detection of seizures requires more electrodes.

electrodes and are abbreviated as C, O, and A, respectively. Each of these letters is followed by a number (1–4) to indicate the side of the electrode; odd numbers (1 or 3) refer to the left side and even numbers (2 or 4) refer to the right side, therefore:

- O_1 and O_2 are the left and right occipital electrodes, respectively.
- A_1 and A_2 are the left and right auricular electrodes, respectively.
- C_3 and C_4 are the left and right central electrodes, respectively.
- To magnify the amplitude (voltage difference) of the EEG signals, the exploring (recording) electrodes are usually referenced to the auricular electrodes of the opposite side (e.g., C_4–A_1 means the right central electrode is the exploring electrode and is referenced to the left auricular electrode; the other electrode pairs will be C_3–A_2, O_1–A_2, and O_2–A_1).
- The EEG in PSG is recorded only from one side while the leads in the opposite side are kept in place as a backup for cases of malfunction of the recoding side while the patient is asleep. Optimal sleep staging requires two exploring electrodes (C and O) but a minimum of one central exploring electrode is needed for definition of sleep stages[75] (central leads are good in capturing most EEG signals as will be discussed later[76, 77]).
- The placement of the EEG leads is explained in Figure 10.1.[78]

EEG Waves[75]

Distinct EEG waves are present and each is differentiated from one another by its frequency in seconds (Hertz or Hz),[†] amplitude, and/or shape. The following are the wave patterns in human sleep; see Figure 10.2a–i.

- Standard wave patterns:
  - *Beta waves* (>13 Hz) are seen when the patient is awake and alert or excited. Beta waves are not seen during sleep; Figure 10.2a.
  - *Alpha waves* (8–13 Hz) are seen when the patient is awake and relaxed. They continue to be seen in stage 1 sleep but with reduced numbers; Figure 10.2b.
  - *Theta waves* (4–7 Hz) are mainly seen in sleep stages 1 and 2; Figure 10.2c.
  - Delta waves (<4 Hz) are seen in sleep stages 3 and 4; Figure 10.2d.

[†] Also referred to as cycles per seconds or cps.

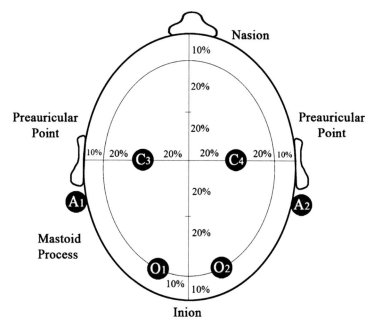

FIGURE 10.1. Schematic of the 10–20 EEG electrode placement system. Landmarks are the nasion (the bridge of the nose), inion (the prominence of the occiput), and the right and left preauricular points. The lines between nasion and inion and between the preauricular points are divided into 10 and 20% segments as shown. The central leads are placed over the preauricular line, 20% from the midline. The occipital leads are placed over an imaginary circle as shown, 10% from the midline. The auricular leads are placed over the mastoid processes.

- Other EEG patterns:
  - *Slow waves* (<2 Hz) represent a slow form of delta waves with high amplitudes (voltage criteria for slow waves: trough to peak is $\geq$75 μV). They are seen in sleep stages 3 and 4; Figure 10.2e.[‡]
  - *Sleep spindles* are oscillations of 12–14 Hz with duration of 0.5–1.5 s.[79] They are seen in stage 2 sleep but may persist into stage 3 and 4; Figure 10.2f.
  - *K complexes (Ks)* are high-altitude, biphasic waves of >0.5-s duration with an initial upward (negative) deflection

---

[‡] Slow waves in older patients may not meet the voltage criteria but are still considered.

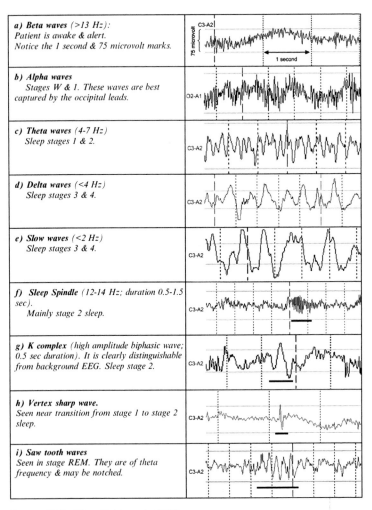

a) Beta waves *(>13 Hz):* Patient is awake & alert. Notice the 1 second & 75 microvolt marks.	
b) Alpha waves Stages W & 1. These waves are best captured by the occipital leads.	
c) Theta waves *(4-7 Hz)* Sleep stages 1 & 2.	
d) Delta waves *(<4 Hz)* Sleep stages 3 & 4.	
e) Slow waves *(<2 Hz)* Sleep stages 3 & 4.	
f) Sleep Spindle *(12-14 Hz; duration 0.5-1.5 sec).* Mainly stage 2 sleep.	
g) K complex *(high amplitude biphasic wave; 0.5 sec duration). It is clearly distinguishable from background EEG.* Sleep stage 2.	
h) Vertex sharp wave. Seen near transition from stage 1 to stage 2 sleep.	
i) Saw tooth waves Seen in stage REM. They are of theta frequency & may be notched.	

FIGURE 10.2. Wave Patterns in EEG.

followed by a downward (positive) deflection[§,¶,75]. A cardinal feature of K complexes is that they are clearly distinguishable from background EEG activity. Sleep spindles may be superimposed on K complexes. Ks are seen in stage 2 sleep (may be seen in stages 3 and 4 but are then indistinguishable from background EEG[75]); Figure 10.2g.

[§] A positive voltage in EEG means a downward deflection and vice versa, a concept that sometimes is referred to as "negative up" rule.

[¶] Slow waves may be thought of as a series of two or more K complexes.[80]

- *Vertex sharp waves* are narrow, high-amplitude negative (upward) waves seen in stage 1 and near transition from stage 1 to stage 2 sleep; Figure 10.2h.
- *Saw-tooth waves* are waves of theta frequency and may be notched. They are seen in stage REM sleep but are not essential for REM definition; Figure 10.2i.[81]
- Alpha waves are best recorded by the occipital leads while the rest of EEG waves (including slow waves, Ks, and spindles) are best recorded by the central leads. This is why the central leads are essential for PSG recording.[76, 77]

Electroocculography

- Is used to record the eye movements, which are essential to define stage REM sleep. Because the eye has a potential difference (cornea is positive with respect to the retina), then measuring this potential (polarity) difference makes it possible to record eye movements using ocular electrodes; Figure 10.3a. These electrodes are placed at the right outer canthus (*ROC*) and the left outer canthus (*LOC*).‖
- Remember that ROC and LOC deflections are out of phase when the eyes move. This phenomenon is used to differentiate true eye movements from artifacts. For example, ocular leads may capture high-voltage EEG signals such as K complexes or slow waves but the deflections recorded at ROC and LOC will be in-phase (same direction) and should not be mistaken for an eye movement; Figure 10.3d.
- As in EEG, to amplify the signals acquired from ROC and LOC, the ocular leads are usually referenced to the opposite auricular leads and abbreviated as ROC-A_1 and LOC-A_2.[**,82]

‖Right and left ocular electrodes are placed at the right outer canthus (ROC) and left outer canthus (LOC), respectively, with the right electrode placed slightly above and the left slightly below the eye level, in order to record vertical eye movements.[75] Keeping the eyeball polarity in mind, moving the eyes to the right will bring the cornea (relatively positive) of the right eye closer to the right ocular lead and the retina (relatively negative) of the left eye closer to the left ocular lead. This will result in a downward (positive) deflection at ROC and an upward (negative) deflection at LOC, which means that the deflections are out of phase (opposite direction). The same thing will happen if the eyes move upward, as the right ocular lead is at a higher level than the left one. The opposite thing should happen if the eyes move to the left or downward; Figure 10.3a.

** Some laboratories reference the ocular leads to the auricular leads in the same side, i.e., ROC-A_2 and LOC-A_1 or to one auricular lead, i.e., ROC-A_2 and LOC A_2.[82]

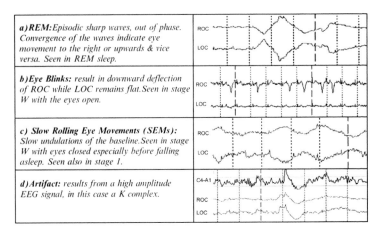

a)REM: *Episodic sharp waves, out of phase. Convergence of the waves indicate eye movement to the right or upwards & vice versa. Seen in REM sleep.*	
b)Eye Blinks: *result in downward deflection of ROC while LOC remains flat. Seen in stage W with the eyes open.*	
c) Slow Rolling Eye Movements (SEMs): *Slow undulations of the baseline. Seen in stage W with eyes closed especially before falling asleep. Seen also in stage 1.*	
d)Artifact: *results from a high amplitude EEG signal, in this case a K complex.*	

FIGURE 10.3. The different eye movements.

- Two distinct eye movements can be recorded through the ocular leads:
  - *REMs* are episodic, sharp waves with a usually flat baseline between movements; Figure 10.3a. REMs are seen typically in stage REM sleep, but similar waves can be seen in stage W with the eyes open representing the normal eye movements. Eye blinks show usually as downward deflections at ROC only; Figure 10.3b.
  - *Slow rolling eye movements* (SEMs) appear as a smooth undulation of the tracing (baseline), Figure 10.3c. These movements are seen in stage W with eyes closed and in stage 1 and disappear in stages 2, 3, and 4.

Chin Electromyography

- The main implication for chin EMG is to help in identifying REM sleep.[75] Three EMG leads are placed at the mental and submental areas and the voltage between two of them is measured. The third lead is reserved for cases of malfunction of any other lead.
- Because the body muscles normally relax during REM sleep, the chin EMG becomes minimal during REM (equal to or lower than the lowest EMG amplitude in NREM sleep). Typically, the chin EMG activity drops with onset of REM sleep. During deep sleep, chin EMG is usually low, but still higher than that of REM sleep. Chin EMG is highest during wakefulness.

Scoring Sleep Stages, Wakefulness, and Arousal

Before discussing the scoring technique, it is important to discuss some concepts of PSG recording and scoring:

Concepts of EEG Recording and Scoring

- Before the era of computerized PSG recording, PSG used to be recorded on paper with a standard paper speed of 10 mm/s.[‡] Currently, computers have made PSG recording and scoring easier with the ability to compress or decompress tracings, enlarge or contract scale, and change the page or tracing format.
- Each 30 s of PSG recording (fit on one screen) represent a distinct time segment termed an *epoch*. Each epoch is divided horizontally into 1-s segments by means of vertical dashed lines to help in distinguishing EEG waves. Longitudinally, because voltage criteria are required to define slow waves, two faint horizontal lines are drawn at the EEG tracing where the distance between them is equivalent to 75 μV. Slow waves have to cross these two lines to meet the voltage criteria, see Figure 10.2a.[‡‡]
- In scoring sleep and wakefulness, each epoch is scored independently and then the scoring of all epochs is added together and presented in the final report. Because an epoch may show more than one stage of sleep, scoring should be according to the predominant stage.
- Remember that the wave frequency reflects the brain activity. Therefore, the frequency is highest when the patient is awake but slows down as the patient gets to sleep and slows down further as he/she goes into deep sleep.

Scoring Sleep Based on EEG, EOG, and Chin EMG[75]

- Stage W (eyes open; patient relaxed):
  - EEG in this stage shows low voltage, high-frequency waves with attenuated alpha activity. EOG may show REMs and blinks, and chin EMG activity is typically increased; Figure 10.4a.
- Stage W (eyes closed; patient drowsy):
  - EEG here consists of low voltage, high-frequency waves with >50% alpha waves/epoch (alpha waves are not attenuated here). EOG shows slow rolling eye movements and chin EMG is increased; Figure 10.4b.

[‡] Paper speed in recording EEG for detection of seizures is slower (15–30 mm/s).

[‡‡] In paper recording, a 50-μV stimulus results in a 1-cm longitudinal deflection. This makes 75-μV equivalent to 1.5-cm deflection.

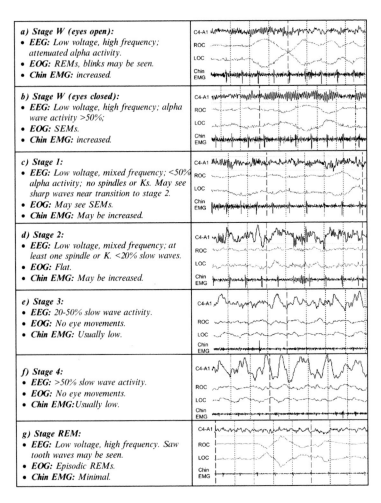

a) Stage W (eyes open): • ***EEG:*** *Low voltage, high frequency;* *attenuated alpha activity.* • ***EOG:*** *REMs, blinks may be seen.* • ***Chin EMG:*** *increased.*	
b) Stage W (eyes closed): • ***EEG:*** *Low voltage, high frequency; alpha* *wave activity >50%;* • ***EOG:*** *SEMs.* • ***Chin EMG:*** *increased.*	

c) Stage 1:
• ***EEG:*** *Low voltage, mixed frequency; <50%*
  alpha activity; no spindles or Ks. May see
  sharp waves near transition to stage 2.
• ***EOG:*** *May see SEMs.*
• ***Chin EMG:*** *May be increased.*	

d) Stage 2: • ***EEG:*** *Low voltage, mixed frequency; at* *least one spindle or K. <20% slow waves.* • ***EOG:*** *Flat.* • ***Chin EMG:*** *May be increased.*	
e) Stage 3: • ***EEG:*** *20-50% slow wave activity.* • ***EOG:*** *No eye movements.* • ***Chin EMG:*** *Usually low.*	
f) Stage 4: • ***EEG:*** *>50% slow wave activity.* • ***EOG:*** *No eye movements.* • ***Chin EMG:*** *Usually low.*	
g) Stage REM: • ***EEG:*** *Low voltage, high frequency. Saw* *tooth waves may be seen.* • ***EOG:*** *Episodic REMs.* • ***Chin EMG:*** *Minimal.*	

FIGURE 10.4. Sleep stages.

• Stage 1 sleep:
  – EEG shows low voltage, mixed frequency waves (alpha and theta) with <50% alpha waves/epoch. Sharp waves may be present near transition to stage 2. Typically, stage 1 does not have sleep spindles or K complexes. EOG continues to show slow rolling eye movement with increased chin EMG activity; Figure 10.4c.

- Stage 2 sleep:
  - EEG here is similar to stage 1 (low voltage, mixed frequency) but it must show at least one sleep spindle or K complex with <20% slow wave activity/epoch. EOG should record no eye movements and chin EMG activity is still increased; Figure 10.4d.
- Stage 3 sleep:
  - EEG should show 20–50% slow wave activity/epoch. EOG shows no eye movements and chin EMG activity usually slows down during this stage; Figure 10.4e.
- Stage 4 sleep:
  - EEG should show >50% slow wave activity/epoch. EOG shows no eye movements and chin EMG activity is usually low; Figure 10.4f.[§§]
- Stage REM sleep:
  - Is identified mainly by the presence of REMs in EOG and minimal activity in chin EMG. EEG shows low voltage, mixed frequency waves with no spindles or Ks (as in stage 1) and may show saw-tooth waves. The presence of saw-tooth waves supports the definition of REM sleep but their absence does not exclude REM; Figure 10.4g.

Additional Rules for Scoring Sleep

- Because sleep spindles and K complexes (in stage 2) and eye movements (in stage REM) are episodic (i.e., are not necessarily seen in every epoch of stage 2 or stage REM, respectively), additional staging rules were introduced concerning these two sleep stages:[75]
  - The 3-min rule for stage 2:
    - (a) *If no arousal is present*: If a period of time between two epochs of unequivocal stage 2 (i.e., containing spindles or Ks) is less than 3 min and the intervening sleep would otherwise meet criteria for stage 1 (<50% alpha activity) with no evidence of intervening arousal, then this period of sleep is scored as stage 2. If that period is ≥3 min, then this period of sleep is scored as stage 1; Figure 10.5a, b.
    - (b) *If arousal is present*: If there is an arousal within the intervening sleep (<3 min), then the epochs following the arousal are scored according to their nature while the

---

[§§] The distinction between sleep stages 3 and 4 is not essential in interpreting PSG and some laboratories score stages 3 and 4 as *deep sleep, delta sleep, or slow wave sleep*.[83]

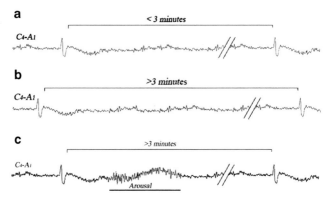

FIGURE 10.5. The 3-min rule for stage 2. (a) Two Ks separated by <3 min without arousal; epochs between the two Ks are staged as stage 2; (b) Two Ks separated by >3 min, so epochs between the two Ks are staged as stage 1; (c) Two Ks separated by <3 min but with an arousal; epochs following arousal are staged according to their nature, in this case stage 1.

epochs before the arousal will still be scored as stage 2; Figure 10.5c.

- The REM rule:
  (a) *If no arousal is present*: If any section of the record is contiguous with an unequivocal stage REM and has a chin EMG and EEG consistent with stage REM, then that section should be scored as stage REM regardless of whether eye movements are present.[¶¶]
  (b) *If arousal is present*, then the distinction is between stage 1 and REM: If the arousal is very brief and/or saw-tooth waves are present following the arousal, then that section is scored as stage REM. If the arousal is prolonged and/or slow rolling eye movements or sharp waves are present following arousal, then that section is scored as stage 1.
  (c) In stage REM sleep, epochs that exhibit REMs are sometimes referred to as *phasic REM* while those that do not exhibit REMs are referred to as *tonic REM*.

Scoring Arousals

- An arousal in NREM sleep is defined as a brief awakening characterized by abrupt shift in EEG frequency, which may include

---

[¶¶] Once a REM sleep is identified, scorer scrolls backward and restudy the previous segment of sleep and rescore it according to this rule.

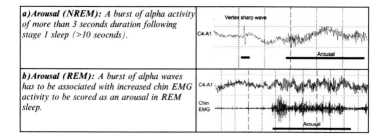

a) Arousal (NREM): A burst of alpha activity of more than 3 seconds duration following stage 1 sleep (>10 seocnds).	Vertex sharp wave C4-A1 Arousal
b) Arousal (REM): A burst of alpha waves has to be associated with increased chin EMG activity to be scored as an arousal in REM sleep.	C4-A1 Chin EMG Arousal

FIGURE 10.6. Arousals.

theta waves, alpha waves, and/or frequencies >16 Hz (usually bursts of alpha waves), lasting 3 s or longer; Figure 10.6a,[III],[84]

- In REM sleep, there must be a concurrent increase in chin EMG activity in addition; Figure 10.6b. This is because bursts of alpha activity are seen normally in REM sleep.[86]

- To be scored as an arousal, such frequency change should be preceded by at least ten continuous seconds of any stage of sleep. Usually there is a rapid return to a pattern consistent with sleep after an arousal, which is mostly the same sleep stage prior to arousal. An awakening, however, is a complete change from any stage of sleep to wakefulness (at least an epoch of stage W). The sleep stage following an awakening can be different from that prior to the awakening.

- The number of arousals per hour of sleep is termed the *arousal index*, which is normally ≤20/h and increases with age.[182] An elevated arousal index is associated with daytime sleepiness.[85, 87]

RESPIRATORY EVENTS

Respiratory events including apnea and hypopnea are scored using airflow, oximetric recording, abdominal and chest movements.

Airflow

- Is measured during PSG in order to detect apneas and hypopneas. Different techniques are used to measure airflow:
  - *Temperature-sensitive devices* are placed close to the nose and mouth to sense the change in temperature of the exhaled air, which is translated into a flow signal in the PSG record. This method is a qualitative method that cannot accurately

---

[III] Another definition of a brief arousal is that of ≥2-s duration with no alteration of sleep stage.[85]

detect the amount of flow and, therefore, makes detection of hypopnea problematic. It may also falsely record airflow during apneic episodes if the transducer touches the body. Two types of such devices are available:

(a) Thermistor: change in temperature results in change in resistance of transducer.[88, 89]

(b) Thermocouple: change in temperature results in change in voltage of transducer.

– *Exhaled CO_2 measurement* by continuously sampling the exhaled air (rich in CO_2) through a nasal/oral cannula connected to a CO_2 analyzer. A time delay is expected for the transfer and analysis of the sampled air. Small expiratory puffs (again rich in CO_2) that may take place during inspiratory apneas may be misinterpreted as airflow by the CO_2 analyzer, which limits the use of this method.

– *Pneumotachography* is an accurate method of measuring airflow but is less comfortable as a mask covering the nose and mouth is needed to measure the pressure difference created by airflow.

– *Nasal pressure* can be measured by a pressure transducer connected to a nasal cannula. This method is convenient and is semiquantitative, which makes it the most popular method.

– *V-sum signal* is derived from chest and abdominal movement; see next session. It is semiquantitative and is sometimes called *effort sum*.[90]

Chest and Abdominal Movements

• Are measured using bands with coils applied around the chest and abdomen. Changes in the inductance (inductance plethysmography) of these coils due to chest and abdominal expansion during inspiration are recorded as deflections in the PSG traces. A computerized summation of the chest and abdominal movement signals is reported as V-sum, which is considered a semiquantitative measurement of tidal volume (airflow); Figure 10.7b. These can be, but are not usually, calibrated for volume displacement.

• Tracings corresponding to airflow, V-sum, chest and abdominal movement are adjusted in such a way that an upward deflection indicates inspiration and a downward deflection indicates expiration.

Pulse Oximetry

• Is used to measure O_2 saturation (S_pO_2) during sleep using a finger or ear probe. Nadir saturation is delayed by 6–8 s due to

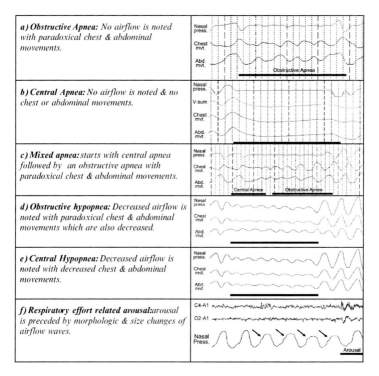

a) Obstructive Apnea: No airflow is noted with paradoxical chest & abdominal movements.	Nasal press. / Chest mvt. / Abd. mvt. — Obstructive Apnea
b) Central Apnea: No airflow is noted & no chest or abdominal movements.	Nasal press. / V-sum / Chest mvt. / Abd. mvt.
c) Mixed apnea: starts with central apnea followed by an obstructive apnea with paradoxical chest & abdominal movements.	Nasal press. / Chest mvt. / Abd. mvt. — Central Apnea / Obstructive Apnea
d) Obstructive hypopnea: Decreased airflow is noted with paradoxical chest & abdominal movements which are also decreased.	Nasal press. / Chest mvt. / Abd. mvt.
e) Central Hypopnea: Decreased airflow is noted with decreased chest & abdominal movements.	Nasal press. / Chest mvt. / Abd. mvt.
f) Respiratory effort related arousal:arousal is preceded by morphologic & size changes of airflow waves.	C4-A1 / O2-A1 / Nasal Press. — Arousal

FIGURE 10.7. Respiratory events.

circulatory and instrumental delay. A desaturation is defined as a drop of S_pO_2 by 4% from the baseline.

Scoring Respiratory Events (Apnea and Hyponea)

- Apnea is defined arbitrarily as absence of airflow (or flattening of V-sum tracing) at the nose and mouth for 10 s or more. Apnea is divided into the following:
  - *Obstructive apnea* is when chest and abdomen move paradoxically (out of phase tracing; Figure 10.7a).
  - *Central apnea* is when no chest or abdominal movements are detected; Figure 10.7b.
  - *Mixed apnea* is when no chest or abdominal movements are detected initially followed by paradoxical movements of the chest and abdomen; Figure 10.7c.

- *Hypopnea* is defined as a reduction in airflow (or V-sum) by a $\frac{1}{2}$[89, 90, 181] or $\frac{2}{3}$[91] from baseline for 10 s or more. Hypopneas are more difficult to detect and some experts mandate the presence of arterial desaturation (a drop S_pO_2 by 4%)[92] together with the reduction in airflow to define hypopnea. Hypopneas can be obstructive or central.
  - *Obstructive hypopnea* is when chest and abdomen move paradoxically; Figure 10.7d.
  - *Central hypopnea* is when chest and abdominal movements continue to be in-phase but with a lower amplitude; Figure 10.7e.

- Apnea and hypopnea are usually followed by an arousal that helps in their identification.

- *Apnea hypopnea index* (AHI) is the average number of apnea and hypopnea per hour of sleep. It is sometimes called the *respiratory disturbance index*. *Apnea index* (AI) and *hypopnea index* (HI) are similarly defined. By consensus, AHI is used to define the severity of sleep apnea (obstructive and central) as follows:
  - <5/h is normal and
  - 5–15/h is mild
  - 15–30/h is moderate and
  - >30/h is severe.

- *Respiratory effort-related arousal* (RERA)[73, 74, 93] is seen in the upper airway resistance syndrome (UARS) and is not associated with apnea or hypopnea (UARS has a normal AHI of <5). RERA is characterized by change in shape and progressive increase in size (width) of the airflow inspiratory waves prior to the, otherwise, unexplained arousals; Figure 10.7f. These changes are typically not associated with a decrease in S_pO_2. The arousals (in the form of bursts of alpha waves) usually last for 3–14 s in UARS. Progressive inversed negative swings in esophageal pressure (using esophageal balloon system during PSG) prior to arousal are considered diagnostic but are not generally employed clinically.

SCORING PERIODIC LIMB MOVEMENTS OF SLEEP

PLMs may be a cause for sleep fragmentation and daytime sleepiness (periodic limb movement disorder or PLMD). It may also take place before sleep onset resulting in sleep onset insomnia as in restless leg syndrome (RLS). PLMs are scored using leg EMG electrodes.

Leg Electromyography

- Right and left EMG leads are placed over the right and left tibialis anterior muscles and the signals acquired are fed to a single recording channel.*** A leg movement will be recorded as a sudden increase in the leg electromyography (leg EMG) activity. For leg movements to be part of PLM of sleep, a sequence of four or more leg movements should be present and each leg movement should be separated from the adjacent leg movements by 5–90s.[180] *The duration of each leg movement should be 0.5–5 s.* The number of PLMs per hour of sleep is the *PLM index* (PLM-I). A PLM-I of <5 is considered normal, 5–25 is mild, 25–50 is moderate, and >50 is severe.[178]
- In PLMD, leg movements may result in arousals, which can be seen in EEG as a burst of alpha waves; Figure 10.8a. These arousals can result in sleep fragmentation and excessive daytime hypersomnolence associated with PLMD. On the other hand, arousals may trigger leg movements, which, in this case, follow the arousals and should not be counted as PLMs.††† *PLM arousal index* (PLM-AI) refers to PLMs accompanied by arousal per hour of sleep. This index is better in defining PLMD than PLM-I as it takes into consideration the arousals caused by PLMs. Severe insomnia and/or excessive daytime sleepiness have been associated with a PLM-AI of >25/h. PLMs usually take place in NREM sleep.

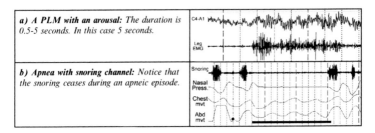

a) A PLM with an arousal: *The duration is 0.5-5 seconds. In this case 5 seconds.*	
b) Apnea with snoring channel: *Notice that the snoring ceases during an apneic episode.*	

FIGURE 10.8. A PLM arousal, snoring.

*** Some labs use a separate channel for each leg EMG tracing. In this case, simultaneous bilateral leg movements are counted as one.

††† Leg movements may be used to help identifying arousals, together with the other parameters.

MISCELLANEOUS PSG CHANNELS

Electrocardiography

- Is used to detect arrhythmias during sleep especially during periods of obstructive apneas/hypopneas. The most important arrhythmias encountered include bradycardias and ventricular asystole lasting longer than 10 s,[94–98] nonsustained SVT and VT, atrial fibrillation,[99, 100] and sinus arrhythmias.

Sleep Position

- Is determined manually (using a video monitor) or using posture detecting devices. Respiratory events related to OSA preferentially take place while in the supine position.

Snoring

- A microphone may be used to record the snoring as a separate channel. This may help to identify sleep onset (when the patient starts snoring at the beginning of the study) and the apneic episodes (snoring tracing disappears when there is no airflow); see Figure 10.8b.

Visual and Auditory Monitoring

- Visual monitoring is done through a low-light video camera to monitor sleep position (as discussed) and to check for parasomnias, which can be easily synchronized with the PSG. Auditory monitoring is required to provide assistance to the patient if needed.

CONCEPTS OF PSG INTERPRETATION

Biocalibration

- Is an essential procedure that should be performed prior to any sleep study (PSG). Its role is to ensure appropriate technical function of the components of the polysomnograph in response to different biological stimuli.
  - *Checking eye movements and blinking*: by asking the patient to keep the head still and look to the left, right, up, and down and then to blink, Figure 10.9a.
  - *Checking EEG*: first with the eyes closed looking for alpha activity (and slow rolling eye movements in the EOG chan-

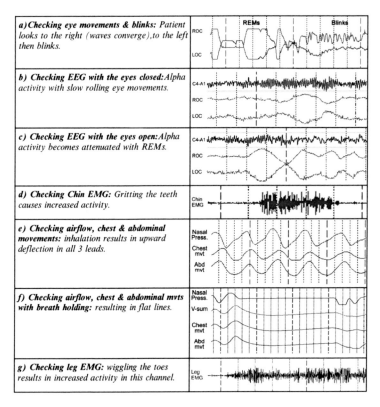

a) *Checking eye movements & blinks:* Patient looks to the right (waves converge),to the left then blinks.	
b) *Checking EEG with the eyes closed:* Alpha activity with slow rolling eye movements.	
c) *Checking EEG with the eyes open:* Alpha activity becomes attenuated with REMs.	
d) *Checking Chin EMG:* Gritting the teeth causes increased activity.	
e) *Checking airflow, chest & abdominal movements:* inhalation results in upward deflection in all 3 leads.	
f) *Checking airflow, chest & abdominal mvts with breath holding:* resulting in flat lines.	
g) *Checking leg EMG:* wiggling the toes results in increased activity in this channel.	

FIGURE 10.9. Biocalibration.

nels) – Figure 10.9b and then with the eyes open looking for attenuation of alpha activity; Figure 10.9c.[‡‡‡]

- *Checking chin EMG:* by asking the patient to grit the teeth and observing an appropriate increase in the chin EMG activity; Figure 10.9d.
- *Checking airflow, chest and abdominal movements:* by asking the patient to inhale and exhale and observing an appropriate deflection of all three channels that should be adjusted so that they have the same polarity with an upward deflection during inhalation, as discussed earlier. The patient is then asked to take a deep breath and then hold to simulate apnea

---

[‡‡‡] Patients who naturally have no or low alpha activity can be identified during biocalibration, which helps anticipating the type of stage 1 sleep in them.

that should be translated as flat lines on these three channels; Figure 10.9e, f.[§§§]

– *Checking leg movements*: by asking the patient to wiggle the right and left toes resulting in appropriately increased leg EMG; Figure 10.9g.

PSG Artifacts

ECG Artifact

• Is a very common and easily recognized artifact. It is made of periodic deflections corresponding to the QRS complexes and resembles them in shape, commonly seen in EEG tracings but can be seen in the other tracings too, as chin EMG and EOG; Figure 10.10a. This artifact is minimized by placing the reference auricular electrode directly over the bone (mastoid process) and avoiding the neck soft tissue, which may conduct the ECG signals. Another way of overcoming this artifact is by referencing the exploring EEG electrode to both auricular electrodes, as positive and negative ECG signals going to each auricular electrode will cancel each other out.

Sixty-Cycle Artifact

• Occurs when a recording electrode is disconnected or has high impedance, which results in recording a 60-Hz AC electrical activity from the power lines instead; Figure 10.10b. This artifact affects mainly the EEG and EOG leads. It can be minimized by proper placement of electrodes and by using certain filters in the AC amplifiers. Switching to another electrode may be necessary.

Sweat Artifact

• Is caused by sweat getting in contact with a recording electrode altering its potential, which results in recording a slow undulation of the baseline activity.[¶¶¶] If EEG electrodes are affected, the undulated baseline may be mistaken for slow

---

[§§§] The patient may be asked to breathe through the mouth, which should show movement of chest and abdominal tracing but not the airflow tracing.

[¶¶¶] If sweat artifact is synchronous (in-phase) with respiration, it is called *respiratory artifact*.

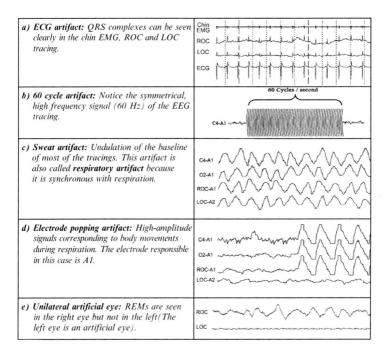

a) ECG artifact: QRS complexes can be seen clearly in the chin EMG, ROC and LOC tracing.	Chin EMG / ROC / LOC / ECG tracings
b) 60 cycle artifact: Notice the symmetrical, high frequency signal (60 Hz) of the EEG tracing.	60 Cycles / second — C4-A1 tracing
*c) Sweat artifact: Undulation of the baseline of most of the tracings. This artifact is also called **respiratory artifact** because it is synchronous with respiration.*	C4-A1 / O2-A1 / ROC-A1 / LOC-A2 tracings
d) Electrode popping artifact: High-amplitude signals corresponding to body movements during respiration. The electrode responsible in this case is A1.	C4-A1 / O2-A1 / ROC-A1 / LOC-A2 tracings
e) Unilateral artificial eye: REMs are seen in the right eye but not in the left (The left eye is an artificial eye).	ROC / LOC tracings

FIGURE 10.10. PSG Artifacts.

delta waves resulting in overestimation of sleep stages 3 and 4. This artifact may be generalized (if patient is sweating heavily) or confined to the side that the patient is lying on. This artifact may be minimized by lowering room temperature, uncovering the patient or using a fan especially in obese patients; Figure 10.10c.

Electrode Popping Artifact

• Is caused by complete loss of signals from one electrode (as complete detachment from the skin or complete dryness of the conducting gel) resulting in high-amplitude signals corresponding to body movement during respiration; Figure 10.10d. The offending electrode can be easily identified by looking for a common lead in the affected channels. It is corrected by switching to an alternative electrode.

Unilateral Artificial Eye

- Results in unilateral deflection of EOG during stage REM sleep leading, if unnoticed, to underestimation of REM sleep; Figure 10.10e. This confusion can be avoided by a proper history taking and a proper biocalibration.

APPROACH TO PSG SCORING

Scoring PSG is the most important part of PSG interpretation, as the final report and ultimately the final diagnosis are largely based on the various scores. A computerized scoring program[100-108] is currently available but does not replace manual scoring. Different approaches for scoring may be followed by which the scorer goes through the study several rounds, scoring different channels. The following is a suggested approach:

- First round is for scoring sleep stages, arousals, and wakefulness: by studying the EEG, EOG, and chin EMG. The sleep architecture and the arousal index can then be determined.
- Second round is for scoring respiratory events: by studying airflow, chest and abdominal movements, V-sum, S_pO_2, and snoring. During this round, the scorer should differentiate central from obstructive events and identify events associated with arousals. AI, HI, and AHI can then be determined. Apneas and hypopneas become easily identified if tracings are compressed so that the computer screen accommodates three epochs at a time (90 s).
- Third round is for scoring leg movements: by studying the leg EMG. The scorer should identify movements that meet the criteria for PLMs and identify those associated with arousals. PLM-I and PLM-AI can then be determined. Consider UARS if arousals are not explained on the bases of respiratory events and PLMs.
- Fourth round is for studying the ECG for arrhythmias especially during a respiratory event.

SLEEP ARCHITECTURE

Definitions

- *Time in bed* (TIB) is the monitoring period (from lights-out to lights-on).||||

||||Lights-out is the point in time at which lights are turned off to allow the patient to sleep; lights-on is when the patient is awakened in the morning.

- *Movement time* refers to epochs in which sleep stage is indeterminate due to movement artifacts.[83, 109]
- *Total sleep time* (TST) is the total minutes of sleep (stages 1–4 and REM).
- *Wake after sleep onset* (WASO) is the minutes of wakefulness after initial sleep onset and before the final awakening. Increased WASO indicates poor sleep efficiency (i.e., sleep fragmentation) and results in daytime hypersomnolence (e.g., sleep-maintenance insomnia).
- *Sleep period time* (SPT) is TST + WASO [also called *total sleep period* (TSP)].
- *Sleep efficiency* (SE) is TST/TIB ratio represented as a percentage.
- *Sleep onset latency* (SOL or sleep latency) is the number of minutes from lights-out to the first epoch of sleep. Prolonged sleep latency (sleep-onset insomnia) may be seen in patients with depression.
- *REM latency* is the number of minutes from sleep onset (not from lights-out) to the first epoch of REM sleep. It is typically reduced in patients with narcolepsy,[110, 111] but can be reduced also in OSA, circadian rhythm disorder, endogenous depression,[112] and withdrawal from REM-suppressing drugs.
- *REM density* is the average number of eye movements (REMs) per unit time.
- *Sleep architecture* is the division of TST among the different sleep stages where sleep stages are represented as percentages of TST (or SPT).
- *Hypnogram or histogram*[109] is a graphic representation of sleep architecture; Figure 10.11.

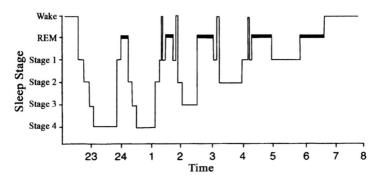

FIGURE 10.11. A histogram, summarizing the normal sleep architecture in a young adult.

Normal Sleep Architecture

- The proportions of sleep stages vary with age and sex; see Table 10.2.[178] Normally, sleep stage 2 is the longest in all age groups and in both sexes representing up to 50% of SPT. Sleep stages 1 and 2 and WASO normally increase with age while deep sleep (stages 3 and 4) decreases with age and becomes predominantly composed of stage 3 sleep. Young people, however, have little stage 3 sleep and their deep sleep is mainly of stage 4; see Table 10.2. Age has little influence on REM sleep.
- The human sleep is normally composed of 3–5 cycles of NREM sleep interrupted by 3–5 cycles of REM sleep. The NREM sleep predominates the first-half of the night while REM sleep predominates the second; Figure 10.11.
- The first cycle of deep sleep starts quickly after sleep onset and is the longest, and gets shorter as sleep progresses. On the other hand, REM sleep occurs every 90–120 min with the first cycle being the shortest and starts late (REM latency of 70–120 min) and the last cycle is the longest, which takes place just before the final awakening. The REM density also increases as sleep progresses; Figure 10.11.[113]
- Because of this composition, parasomnias of deep sleep (such as somnambulism) usually occur during the early hours of sleep while parasomnias of REM sleep (nightmares) are more common in the early morning hours.
- During REM sleep, several unique physiologic changes take place in the body:
  - Most dreams (including nightmares) take place during REM sleep.
  - Skeletal muscle hypotonia: develops during REM sleep to prevent the acting out of dreams. Patients with REM behavior disorder have abnormalities of this protective mechanism and they may have violent behavior.

TABLE 10.2. Sleep architecture in the young, elder, and OSA

	Normal sleep (% SPT)		OSA (% SPT)
	Age 20	Age 60	
Wake	1	8	10
Stage 1	5	10	25
Stage 2	45	57	55
Stage 3 and 4	21	2	0
Stage REM	28	23	10

- Hypotonia of upper airway muscles: results in upper airway obstruction during REM in vulnerable patients leading to OSA. This is why obstructive apneas take place preferentially during REM.[114]
- Ventilatory irregularity: takes place during the phasic REM sleep (REM with eye movements) and results in a reduction in tidal volume (V_T).**** Additionally, there is reduced ventilatory response to hypoxemia and hyprecapnia during REM sleep.[115, 116] Patients with underlying lung disorders experience the most severe O_2 desaturation during the early morning hours, that is when phasic REM is most pronounced. All of the ventilatory muscles except the diaphragm become inactive in REM and hence the hypoventilation and arterial oxygen desaturation.
- Nocturnal penile tumescence takes place during REM sleep.[117]
- Thermoregulatory mechanisms are almost totally shut down during REM sleep.[118]

Final PSG Report

Components of the Final Report

- The final report summarizes the findings of PSG after scoring and can be presented in both numerical and graphic forms. The numerical form contains the following:
  - Sleep architecture: includes TSP, SPT, SE, SOL, number of REM periods, and REM latency. A sleep stage summary is presented in the form of WASO and the different sleep stages which are expressed as percentages of TST or SPT.
  - PLM summary: including PLM index and PLM-AI.
  - Apnea and hypopnea analyses that present AI, HI, and AHI, number of central, obstructive, and mixed events, number of events during REM and NREM sleep, number of events associated with arousals and number of events in relation to position (supine and nonsupine).
  - S_pO_2 summary: showing the different levels of S_pO_2 during stage W, NREM, and REM sleep.
- The graphic form is usually composed of five sections with the time represented on the X-axis. This form includes a hypnogram

---

**** Diaphragm becomes the only active inspiratory muscle during phasic REM.

combined with respiratory events' summary, S_pO_2 tracing, body position and PLMs; Figure 10.12. The presence of a hypnogram allows identifying events in relation to sleep stages.

Interpretation of the Final Report

- The following is a suggested approach:
  - Identify the patient's demographics.
  - Go through the patient's complaints, past history, and current medications.
  - Identify the indication for PSG.
  - Examine sleep architecture and sleep stages by checking SE, TST, and REM [to make sure that the patient had a period of sleep long enough to make a diagnosis (including enough REM)].[††††]
  - Examine the respiratory events during sleep:
    - AHI – to score degree of sleep apnea if present. Check number of events in relation to the following:
      (a) REM (in OSA, events are more common during REM)
      (b) Position (in OSA, events are more likely to be in supine position)
      (c) Identify if events are predominantly obstructive (OSA) or central (CSA).

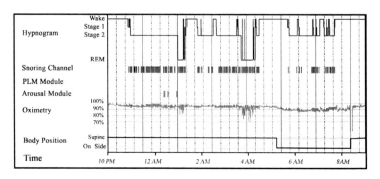

FIGURE 10.12. The final report summarized in this graphic form. Notice that most respiratory events and desaturations occur during REM sleep and while the patient is supine.

[††††] It is hard to pinpoint a minimum duration of sleep sufficient enough to make a confident diagnosis from a PSG. We suggest a minimum duration (TST) of 3 h with at least 10% of REM sleep.

- Study the AI and HI in a similar way as AHI.
- Study S_pO_2 that is best made by looking at the graphic tracing.
  - Examine ECG monitoring comments (made by the scorer) to report any arrhythmias associated with respiratory events.
  - Examine PLM-AI; a high index (>5/h) is suggestive of PLMD (PLM-AI of >25/h is consistent with the diagnosis of PLMD). An elevated PLM index with a normal PLM-AI is suggestive of PLM of sleep, which is not associated with sleep fragmentation and, therefore, daytime sleepiness.

Other Forms of Overnight Sleep Studies

C-PAP Titration PSG

- After prescription of C-PAP in patients with confirmed OSA, C-PAP titration PSG is commonly done to detect the appropriate C-PAP pressure.
- The procedure is similar to the diagnostic PSG except that the patient uses C-PAP machine during the study. Different C-PAP pressures are applied throughout the night and the pressure that best controls the respiratory events is then selected as the appropriate pressure for the patient. The pressure should be adequate to resolve sleep apnea including the respiratory events taking place during REM sleep in the supine position.
- A follow-up study may be performed to assess the adequacy of the initially selected pressure particularly with return of symptoms of OSA (i.e., snoring and daytime sleepiness).

Split Night PSG

- The night is divided into two parts: a diagnostic PSG is done in the first part and a C-PAP titration PSG is done in the second part. Although less costly, it may influence accuracy of PSG as the duration and quality of the diagnostic PSG are reduced. Additionally, the patient's sleep is interrupted as he/she is awakened for application of C-PAP. Finally, the time reserved for C-PAP titration may be insufficient for adequate results.

Auto C-PAP Titration

- An auto C-PAP (smart) machine is capable of automatically changing C-PAP pressure according to patient needs. The PAP data are recoded throughout the night and can be downloaded to a computer. The pressure that the auto C-PAP machine delivered the most during the night is the pressure that is most likely optimal for the patient.

Limited Channel Sleep Studies (Portable Monitoring Devices)[119]

- Sleep studies can be done with fewer channels than the standard PSG, making these studies less expensive and more portable (can be done in the home). At the same time, these studies are less informative but they can still be useful with appropriate patient selection. For the sake of classification, sleep studies are categorized into four types:
  - Type 1: it is the standard PSG with a minimum of 12 channels, as described earlier. This is not a limited channel study and has to be done under supervision in a sleep laboratory.
  - Type 2: minimum of seven channels, including EEG, EOG, chin EMG, ECG or heart rate, airflow, respiratory effort, and S_pO_2.
  - Type 3: minimum of four channels, including ventilation or airflow (at least two channels of respiratory movement, or respiratory movement and airflow), heart rate or ECG, and S_pO_2.
  - Type 4: most monitors of this type measure a single parameter or two parameters, e.g., overnight oximetry, which is the most popular type 4 method.
- These studies can be attended (by a technician) or unattended, full night or split-night, or can be of limited duration (<6 h). Interpretation of type 3 and 4 studies should be done with caution as they cannot score sleep. Certain guidelines are currently available to guide the use of these limited sleep studies.[119]

OVERNIGHT OXIMETRY

Introduction

- Overnight oximetry is a widely used tool for diagnostic and screening purposes for sleep apnea. It is simple, inexpensive,[120] and readily available as a portable test. It is considered a type 4 sleep study because it monitors two variables: S_pO_2 and heart rate.
- Overnight oximetry is usually done in the home‡‡‡‡ as it is simple and can easily be set up by the patient. The data are

---

‡‡‡‡ Overnight oximetry is done sometimes for inpatients if admitted for unrelated issues and are found incidentally to have OSA clinically.

recorded in a recording card and the results can be downloaded and analyzed electronically. The results are usually presented as numerical and graphic forms.

– Numerically, the single most important figure is the oxygen desaturation index (ODI), which is defined as the number of desaturation events per hour. A desaturation event in a respiratory sleep disorder is defined as a reduction in S_pO_2 by $\geq 4\%$ from baseline.[121–125] Other numerical data include the highest, the lowest, and the mean S_pO_2 and heart rate.

– Graphically, data are plotted as saturation and heart rate vs. time; Figure 10.13.

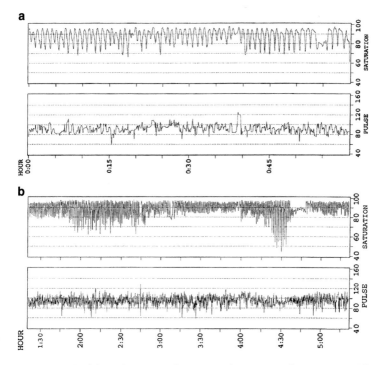

FIGURE 10.13. (a) A 1-h tracing of an overnight oximetry for a patient with severe OSA (ODI: 63/h). Notice the significant desaturations accompanied by significant variation in heart rate. (b) A compressed (4 h) tracing of the same overnight oximetry shown in (a) showing the typical appearance of S_pO_2 and heart rate in a positive test. Notice the significant desaturations that reached critical levels (<50%) at 4:30 AM, which may suggest that the patient was in REM sleep during that event.

Interpretation

- Oxygen desaturation index (ODI):
  - Is normally less than five events per hour.[121, 124–127] ODI cutoff point for the diagnosis of OSA is not well defined. Generally, with an ODI of ≥15/h,[§§§§] the interpreter is more confident to consider a study positive.[128–132] Some laboratories, however, use 5 or 10 events/h as the threshold and all of these values are supported by evidence.[121, 124–127, 133, 134] ODI alone is not sufficient to make a useful conclusion from an overnight oximetric study, as it has to be combined with graphic changes.[135, 136]
- Graphically:
  - In OSA, S_pO_2 drops gradually during an obstructive event but returns rapidly to the baseline when the obstructive event is terminated (e.g., by arousal). This phenomenon is responsible for the saw-tooth waveform pattern of S_pO_2 if plotted against time; Figure 10.14.[137, 138] This wave pattern combined with a high ODI (>15/h) is considered diagnostic in the presence of the appropriate clinical scenario.[127, 137]
  - Central apneas, especially when part of Cheyne-Stokes respiration, produce more symmetrical waveform as the breathing

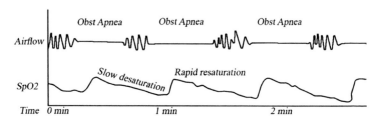

FIGURE 10.14. The characteristic saw-tooth pattern of S_pO_2 in OSA. Notice the slow desaturation and the rapid resaturation. Notice also that there is a delay in the nadir saturation in relation to airflow, which is due to circulatory and instrumental delay (Modified from Netzer et al.[137] With permission.).

---

§§§§ An ODI of 10 is widely used as the cutoff point, which, if used, increases the sensitivity but may not significantly change the specificity if compared to an ODI of 15.

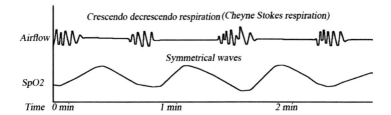

FIGURE 10.15. In CSA (Cheyne-Stokes respiration), S_pO_2 produces more regular and symmetrical waveform due to the regular crescendo–decrescendo pattern of respiration (Modified from Netzer et al.[137] With permission.).

pattern here is more regular (crescendo–decrescendo pattern) compared to that of OSA; Figure 10.15.[137, 138] Central apneas may produce the saw-tooth pattern as well, especially if not associated with Cheyne-Stokes respiration.[137]

- The overlap syndrome¶¶¶¶ may be differentiated from OSA by the duration of the desaturations, being much longer in the overlap syndrome.[139, 140]
- The heart rate response typically shows reflex bradycardias that develop during obstructive events (apneas or hypopneas) in relation to the nadir negative intrathoracic pressure. The heart rate rapidly increases when an obstructive event is terminated; Figure 10.13. Central apneas are not generally associated with this pattern of heart rate response.

Reliability of Overnight Oximetry

- Overnight oximetry is most useful when the clinical index of suspicion for OSA is high. The sensitivity and specificity of overnight oximetry is 100% and 95%, respectively, in patients with AHI of ≥25 events/h, but these values decreased to 75% and 86%, respectively, in patients with AHI of ≥15 events/h.‖‖‖‖[127] This indicates that oximetry is an effective tool for screening patients with moderate-to-severe OSA.[127] It is often difficult to differentiate central from obstructive events with oximetry.
- On the other hand, overnight oximetry has less diagnostic value in patients with mild OSA; these patients will often require full diagnostic PSG.[125] Figure 10.16 presents a reasonable approach to properly utilize overnight oximetry.[137]

¶¶¶¶ The overlap syndrome refers to the coexistence of OSA and COPD.
‖‖‖‖ Other studies showed similar sensitivities and specificities.[128–133,141–149]

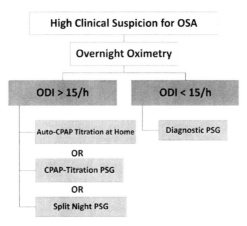

FIGURE 10.16. Approach to patients with strong clinical suspicion for OSA using overnight oximetry as an initial diagnostic study (Modified from Netzer et al.[137] With permission.).

- In conclusion, overnight oximetry can be a useful diagnostic test. It is also a very cost-effective test[120, 125, 150, 151] if utilized appropriately.****

ASSESSMENT OF DAYTIME SLEEPINESS[#]

Multiple Sleep Latency Test

Preparation

- Multiple sleep latency test (MSLT) is useful to assess conditions with excessive somnolence, particularly narcolepsy. The aim of this test is to measure the tendency to fall asleep during the day by measuring the sleep and the REM latencies, which are abnormally short in narcolepsy. The following are important points in preparation for MSLT:
  - MSLT should be preceded by a PSG (usually done on the night that precedes the day of the test) to exclude conditions

----

**** False negative oximetries occur mostly in nonobese patients or in those with short duration apneas. In the case of thin patients, FRC (O_2 reserve) is preserved and O_2 consumption is reduced compared with obese patients.

[#] Tests used to assess daytime sleepiness are done during the day as opposed to PSG that is done at night to assess sleep efficiency.

(e.g., OSA) that may affect sleep architecture and may cause REM-sleep fragmentation resulting in increased REM score in the MSLT. Therefore, the presence of OSA makes the interpretation of the MSLT difficult indicating that sleep apnea should be properly treated first (e.g., with CPAP). A repeat PSG while on CPAP prior to the MSLT is important to ensure that OSA is well controlled before testing. PSG can detect PLMD, which may have the same effect on MSLT as OSA. A PSG is also useful to ensure that the patient slept adequately the night before.

– A 1–2-week sleep diary is important to document the sleep pattern as MSLT results may be affected by lack of adequate sleep in any of the preceding seven nights.[152–156]

– Medications that are known to affect sleep or REM latency[†††††] should be stopped (if possible) at least 2 weeks prior to MSLT. MSLT results are influenced by the chronic or acute usage or acute withdrawal of these drugs. Urine drug screening may be needed in suspected cases.

– Avoidance of alcohol and caffeine on the day of the test is required. Acute withdrawal from high doses of caffeine is prohibited.

Procedure

• MSLT requires only the monitoring of EEG, EOG, and chin EMG for sleep staging. The patient should dress in comfortable street clothes and the test should be performed in a comfortable, dark, and quiet room with appropriate temperature. The patient is then allowed to nap 4–5 times throughout the day, 2 h apart and 1.5–3 h after a normal PSG.

• The patient is given 20 min to fall asleep after lights-out and once asleep an additional 15 min to reach REM sleep. Recordings should be monitored closely by an experienced technologist.

• Naps are terminated if patient:
  – Fails to initiate sleep in 20 min.
  – Fails to reach REM sleep in 15 min after 1st epoch of sleep.
  – Achieved one epoch of unequivocal REM sleep.

Interpretation

• The normal mean sleep latency during MSLT is 10–20 min,[160–167] which decreases with any dyssomnia, mainly OSA. A sleep

---

[†††††] Drugs that affect sleep latency include sedatives, hypnotics, antihistamines and stimulants; drugs that affect REM latency include tricyclic antidepressants, monoamine oxidase inhibitors, lithium, selective serotonin reuptake inhibitors (SSRIs), and amphetamines.[157–159]

latency of <5 min is pathological[160] and associated with impaired functional performance.[153, 155, 168, 169] A sleep latency of 5–10 min is a diagnostic gray area[170] but may be considered mild sleepiness.

- Short sleep latency during the night is considered normal. During the day, sleep latency varies, being shortest near noon or early afternoon (third or fourth nap) and longest during the late afternoon (fifth nap).[162]
- Scoring 0–1 REM periods per five naps is seen in normal individuals but two or more REM periods are diagnostic for narcolepsy.[‡‡‡‡, 161, 166] Sleep-onset REM is seen in 10–15% of patients with narcolepsy[173] but may indicate chronic sleep disturbance[174] or coexistence of OSA and narcolepsy.[175, 176] MSLT should be repeated after the coexisting condition is properly treated.

Maintenance of Wakefulness Test

- Maintenance of wakefulness test (MWT) is used to test the ability to stay awake during the day. It is primarily designed as a measure of safety in occupations dependent on alertness although this test measures wakefulness, not alertness.
- Unlike MSLT, patients here are encouraged to resist sleep for 40 min while seated upright in a bed in a dark, quiet room. The patient is monitored by EEG, EOG, and chin EMG for detection of sleep. The test is terminated if sleep is detected or after 40 min if patient remains awake. This test is then repeated 4–5 times throughout the day.
- The normal MWT latency is 19 min, which is reduced in case of dyssomnias including OSA and narcolepsy. MWT latency increases significantly when these conditions are treated.
- Patients undergoing this test should provide a 1–2 weeks sleep diary and should be off medications or beverages that influence sleep.

Subjective Tests

Epworth Sleepiness Scale[177]

- Is the most popular subjective method of assessing daytime sleepiness. It represents an eight-statement questionnaire that aims at the detection of the degree of the daytime sleepiness over the last month; Table 10.3. Scoring 3–6/24 is considered normal. Scoring 7–9 indicates mild daytime sleepiness and

---

‡‡‡‡ ≥2 REM/4 or 5 naps may be seen in patients with OSA, psychological disorders, or acute withdrawal of REM-suppressing drugs [e.g., tricyclic antidepressants (TCA), Li, SSRI].[165,171,172]

TABLE 10.3. Epworth sleepiness scale

In the last 30 days, how likely are you to doze off or fall asleep in the following situations (in contrast to feeling just tired)? This refers to your usual way of life in recent times. Even if you have not done some of these things recently try to work out how they would have affected you.

0 = would never doze.
1 = slight chance of dozing.
2 = moderate chance of dozing.
3 = high chance of dozing.

Situations:

1. Sitting & reading ( )
2. Watching TV ( )
3. Sitting inactive in a public place ( )
4. As a passenger in a car for an hour without a break ( )
5. Lying down to rest in the afternoon ( )
6. Sitting and talking to someone ( )
7. Sitting quietly after lunch with no alcohol ( )
8. In a car while stopped for a few minutes in traffic ( )

Total score out of 24: ( )

TABLE 10.4. Stanford sleepiness scale

Circle the one number that best describes your level of alertness or sleepiness right now.

1. Feeling active, vital, alert, wide awake.
2. Functioning at a high level but not at peak, able to concentrate.
3. Relaxed, awake but not fully alert, responsive.
4. A little foggy, let down.
5. Foggy, beginning to lose track, difficulty in staying awake.
6. Sleepy, woozy, prefer to lie down.
7. Almost in reverie, cannot stay awake, sleep onset appears imminent.

scoring ≥10/24 indicates moderate to severe sleepiness. Scoring 24/24 indicates an extraordinary sleepiness while scoring 0/24 suggests a hyperarousable or insomniac patient.

Stanford Sleepiness Scale[179]

- Represents a series of statements to the subject who is required to check the one statement that most accurately describes the current state of sleepiness. It is less widely used as it is less specific and relates only to the state of the patient at the time the test is filled. Scoring 1–2 is considered normal and the more you score, the more sleepy you are; Table 10.4.

References

1. Diagnostic Classification Steering Committee, Thopy MJ. International classification of sleep disorders: diagnostic and coding manual. American Sleep Disorders Association, Rochester, NM, 1990.
2. Pack AI. Obstructive sleep apnea. Adv Intern Med 1994;39:517.
3. Young T, Palta M, Dempsey J, et al. The occurrence of sleep-disordered breathing among middle-aged adults. N Engl J Med 1993;328:1230.
4. Parish JM, Somers VK. Obstructive sleep apnea and cardiovascular disease. Mayo Clin Proc 2004;79:1036.
5. Hla KM, Young TB, Bidwell T, et al. Sleep apnea and hypertension: a population based study. Ann Intern Med 1994;120:382.
6. Lavie P, Herer P, Hoffstein V. Obstructive sleep apnoea syndrome as a risk factor for hypertension: population study. BMJ 2000;320:479.
7. Nieto FJ, Young TB, Lind BK, et al. Association of sleep-disordered breathing, sleep apnea, and hypertension in a large community-based study. Sleep Heart Health Study. JAMA 2000;283:1829.
8. Young T, Poppard P, Palta M, et al. Population-based study of sleep-disordered breathing as a risk factor for hypertension. Arch Intern Med 1997;157:1746.
9. Grote L, Ploch T, Heitmann J. Sleep-related breathing disorder is an independent risk factor for systemic hypertension. Am J Respir Crit Care Med 1999;160:1875.
10. Bixler EO, Vgontzas AN, Lin HM, et al. Association of hypertension and sleep-disordered breathing. Arch Intern Med 2000;160:2289.
11. Marin JM, Carrizo SJ, Vicente E, Agusti AG. Long-term cardiovascular outcomes in men with obstructive sleep apnoea-hypopnoea with or without treatment with continuous positive airway pressure: an observational study. Lancet 2005;365:1046.
12. Olson LG, King MT, Hensley MJ, Saunders NA. A community study of snoring and sleep-disordered breathing: health outcomes. Am J Respir Crit Care Med 1995;152:717.
13. Koskenvuo M, Partinen M, Sarna S, et al. Snoring as a risk factor for hypertension and angina pectoris. Lancet 1985;1:893.
14. Schmidt-Nowara WW, Coultas DB, Wiggins C, et al. Snoring in a Hispanic-American population: risk factors and association with hypertension and other morbidity. Arch Intern Med 1990;150:597.
15. Hung J, Whitford EG, Parsons RW, Hillman DR. Association of sleep apnoea with myocardial infarction in men. Lancet 1990;336:261.
16. Arzt M, Young T, Finn L, et al. Association of sleep-disordered breathing and the occurrence of stroke. Am J Respir Crit Care Med 2005;172:1447.
17. Simantirakis EN, Schiza SI, Marketou ME, et al. Severe bradyarrhythmias in patients with sleep apnoea: the effect of continuous positive airway pressure treatment: a long-term evaluation using an insertable loop recorder. Eur Heart J 2004;25:1070.
18. Tilkian AG, Guilleminault C, Schroeder JS, et al. Sleep induced apnea syndrome – prevalence of cardiac arrhythmias and their reversal after tracheostomy. Am J Med 1977;63:348.

19. Miller WP. Cardiac arrhythmias and conduction disturbances in the sleep apnea syndrome. Prevalence and significance. Am J Med 1982;73:317.
20. Zwillich C, Devlin T, White D, Douglas N. Bradycardia during sleep apnea. Characteristics and mechanism. J Clin Invest 1982;69:1286.
21. Alonso-Fernandez A, Garcia-Rio F, Racionero MA, et al. Cardiac rhythm disturbances and ST-segment depression episodes in patients with obstructive sleep apnea-hypopnea syndrome and its mechanisms. Chest 2005;127:15.
22. Gami AS, Friedman PA, Chung MK, et al. Therapy insight: interactions between atrial fibrillation and obstructive sleep apnea. Nat Clin Pract Cardiovasc Med 2005;2:145.
23. Yaggi HK, Concato J, Kernan WN, et al. Obstructive sleep apnea as a risk factor for stroke and death. N Engl J Med 2005;353:2034.
24. Reichmuth KJ, Austin D, Skatrud JB, Young T. Association of sleep apnea and type II diabetes: a population-based study. Am J Respir Crit Care Med 2005;172:1590.
25. Borgel J, Sanner BM, Bittlinsky A, et al. Obstructive sleep apnoea and its therapy influence high-density lipoprotein cholesterol serum levels. Eur Respir J 2006;27:121.
26. Bradley TD, Rutherford R, Grossman RF, et al. Role of daytime hypoxemia in the pathogenesis of right heart failure in the obstructive sleep apnea syndrome. Am Rev Respir Dis 1985;131:835.
27. Sajkov D, Cowie RJ, Thornton AT, et al. Pulmonary hypertension and hypoxemia in obstructive sleep apnea syndrome. Am J Respir Crit Care Med 1994;149:416.
28. Guidry UC, Mendes LA, Evans et al. Echocardiographic features of the right heart in sleep-disordered breathing: the Framingham Heart Study. Am J Respir Crit Care Med 2001;164:933.
29. Arias MA, Garcia-Rio F, Alonso-Fernandez A, et al. Pulmonary hypertension in obstructive sleep apnoea: effects of continuous positive airway pressure: a randomized, controlled cross-over study. Eur Heart J 2006;27:1106.
30. Horne J, Reyner L. Sleep related vehicle accidents. BMJ 1995;310:565.
31. Masa JF, Rubio M, Findley LJ. Habitually sleepy drivers have a high frequency of automobile crashes associated with respiratory disorders during sleep. Am J Respir Crit Care Med 2000;162:1407.
32. Sleep apnea, sleepiness, and driving risk. American Thoracic Society. Am J Respir Crit Care Med 1994;150:1463.
33. Javaheri S, Parker TJ, Liming JD, et al. Sleep apnea in 81 ambulatory male patients with stable heart failure: types and their prevalences, consequences, and presentations. Circulation 1998;97:2154.
34. Javaheri S, Parker TJ, Wexler L, et al. Occult sleep-disordered breathing in stable congestive heart failure. Ann Intern Med 1995;122:487.
35. Dowdell WT, Javaheri S, McGinnis W. Cheyne-Stokes respiration presenting as sleep apnea syndrome. Clinical and polysomnographic features. Am Rev Respir Dis 1990;141:871.

36. Ohayon MM, Priest RG, Zulley J, et al. Prevalence of narcolepsy symptomatology and diagnosis in the European general population. Neurology 2002;58:1826.

37. Ohayon MM, Priest RG, Zulley J, et al. Prevalence of narcolepsy symptomatology and diagnosis in the European general population. Neurology 2002;58:1826.

38. Silber MH, Krahn LE, Olson EJ, Pankratz VS. The epidemiology of narcolepsy in Olmsted County, Minnesota: a population-based study. Sleep 2002;25:197.

39. Okun ML, Lin L, Pelin Z, et al. Clinical aspects of narcolepsy-cataplexy across ethnic groups. Sleep 2002;25:27.

40. Ekbom KA. Restless legs syndrome. Neurology 1960;10:868.

41. O'Keeffe ST, Gavin K, Lavan JN. Iron status and restless leg syndrome in the elderly. Age Ageing 1994;23:200.

42. Earley CJ, Connor JR, Beard JL, et al. Abnormalities in CSF concentrations of ferritin and transferrin in restless legs syndrome. Neurology 2000;54:1698.

43. Allen RP, Barker PB, Wehrl F, et al. MRI measurement of brain iron in patients with restless legs syndrome. Neurology 2001;56:263.

44. Silber MH, Richardson JW. Multiple blood donations associated with iron deficiency in patients with restless legs syndrome. Mayo Clin Proc 2003;78:52.

45. Connor JR, Boyer PJ, Menzies SL, et al. Neuropathological examination suggests impaired brain iron acquisition in restless legs syndrome. Neurology 2003;61:304.

46. Connor JR, Wang XS, Patton SM, et al. Decreased transferrin receptor expression by neuromelanin cells in restless legs syndrome. Neurology 2004;62:1563.

47. Walker S, Fine A, Kryger MH. Sleep complaints are common in a dialysis unit. Am J Kidney Dis 1995;26:751.

48. Thorp ML. Restless legs syndrome. Int J Artif Organs 2001;24:755.

49. Kavanagh D, Siddiqui S, Geddes CC. Restless legs syndrome in patients on dialysis. Am J Kidney Dis 2004;43:43.

50. Harris DC, Chapman JR, Stewart KH, et al. Low dose erythropoietin in maintenance haemodialysis: improvement in quality of life and reduction in true cost of haemodialysis. Aust N Z J Med 1991;21:693.

51. Sloand JA, Shelly MA, Feigin A, et al. A double-blind, placebo-controlled trial of intravenous iron dextran therapy in patients with ESRD and restless legs syndrome. Am J Kidney Dis 2004;43:663.

52. Collado-Seidel V, Kohnen R, Samtleben W, et al. Clinical and biochemical findings in uremic patients with and without restless legs syndrome. Am J Kidney Dis 1998;31:132.

53. O'Hare JA, Abuaisha F, Geoghegan M. Prevalence and forms of neuropathic morbidity in 800 diabetics. Ir J Med Sci 1994;163:132.

54. Lopes LA, Lins Cde M, Adeodato VG, et al. Restless legs syndrome and quality of sleep in type 2 diabetes. Diabetes Care 2005;28:2633.

55. Muller-Felber W, Landgraf R, Wagner S, et al. Follow-up study of sensory-motor polyneuropathy in type 1 (insulin-dependent) diabetic

subjects after simultaneous pancreas and kidney transplantation and after graft rejection. Diabetologia 1991;34 Suppl 1:S113.

56. Garcia-Borreguero D, Odin P, Serrano C. Restless legs syndrome and PD: a review of the evidence for a possible association. Neurology 2003;61:S49.

57. Boyer P, Ondo W, Allen R. Neuropathologic evaluation of the central nervous system in restless legs syndrome: case report and review of the literature. Soc Neurosci 2000;2:2060 (abstract).

58. Krishnan PR, Bhatia M, Behari M. Restless legs syndrome in Parkinson's disease: a case-controlled study. Mov Disord 2003;18:181.

59. Lang AE, Johnson K. Akathisia in idiopathic Parkinson's disease. Neurology 1987;37:477.

60. Tan EK, Lum SY, Wong MC. Restless legs syndrome in Parkinson's disease. J Neurol Sci 2002;196:33.

61. Comella CL, Goetz CG. Akathisia in Parkinson's disease. Mov Disord 1994;9:545.

62. Poewe W, Hogl B. Akathisia, restless legs and periodic limb movements in sleep in Parkinson's disease. Neurology 2004;63:S12.

63. Ekbom KA. Restless legs syndrome. Acta Med Scan Suppl 1945;158:4.

64. Goodman JD, Brodie C, Ayida GA. Restless leg syndrome in pregnancy. BMJ 1988;297:1101.

65. Suzuki K, Ohida T, Sone T, et al. The prevalence of restless legs syndrome among pregnant women in Japan and the relationship between restless legs syndrome and sleep problems. Sleep 2003;26:673.

66. Manconi M, Govoni V, De Vito A, et al. Restless legs syndrome and pregnancy. Neurology 2004;63:1065.

67. Salih AM, Gray RE, Mills KR, Webley M. A clinical serological and neurophysiological study of restless legs syndrome in rheumatoid arthritis. Br J Rheumatol 1994;33:60.

68. Gudbjornsson B, Broman JE, Hetta J, Hallgren R. Sleep disturbances in patients with primary Sjögren's syndrome. Br J Rheumatol 1993;32:1072.

69. Yunus MB, Aldag JC. Restless legs syndrome and leg cramps in fibromyalgia syndrome: a controlled study. BMJ 1996;312:1339.

70. Ondo W, Tan EK, Mansoor J. Rheumatologic serologies in secondary restless legs syndrome. Mov Disord 2000;15:321.

71. Kanter AH. The effect of sclerotherapy on restless legs syndrome. Dermatol Surg 1995;21:328.

72. Earley CJ. Clinical practice. Restless legs syndrome. N Engl J Med 2003;348:2103.

73. Guilleminault C, Stoohs R, Clerk A, et al. A cause of excessive daytime sleepiness. The upper airway resistance syndrome. Chest 1993;104:781–787.

74. Guilleminault C, Stoohs R, Kim Y, et al. Upper airway sleep-disordered breathing in women. Ann Intern Med 1995;122:493–501.

75 Rechtschaffen A, Kales A, eds. A Manual of Standardized Terminology: Techniques and Scoring System for Sleep Stages of Human Subjects. UCLA Brain Information Service/Brain Research Institute, Los Angeles, 1968.

76. Blake H, Gerard RW, Kleitman N. Factors influencing brain potentials during sleep. J Neurophysiol 1939;2:48–60.

77 Brazier MAB. The electrical fields at the surface of the head during sleep. Electroencephalogr Clin Neurophysiol 1949;195–204.

78. Jasper HH. The ten twenty electrode system of the International Federation. Electroencephalogr Clin Neurophysiol 1958;10:371–375.

79. DiPerri R, Meduri M, DiRosa AE, Simone F. Sleep spindles in healthy people. I. Quantitative, automatic analysis in young adult subjects. Boll Soc Ital Biol Sper 1977;53:983–989.

80. Van Leeuwen S. Proposal for an EEG terminology by the terminology committee of the International Federation for Electroencephalography and Clinical Neurophysiology. Electroencephalogr Clin Neurophysiol 1966;20:293–304.

81. Berger RJ, Olley P, Oswald I. The EEG, eye movements and dreams of the blind. QJ Exp Psychol 1962;14:182–186.

82. Carskadon MA. Basics for polygraphic monitoring of sleep. In: Guilleminault C, ed. Sleeping and Waking Disorders: Indications and Techniques. Addison-Wesley, Menlo Park, CA, 1982;1–16.

83. Kryger MH, Thomas R, William CD. Principle and Practice of Sleep Medicine, Second Edition. Saunders, Philadelphia, PA, 1994.

84. American Sleep Disorders Association – The Atlas Task Force. EEG arousals: scoring rules and examples. Sleep 1992;15:174–184.

85. Carskadon MA, Brown ED, Dement WC. Sleep fragmentation in the elderly: relationship to daytime sleep tendency. Neurobiol Aging 1982;3:321–327.

86. Johnson LC, Nute C, Austin MT, Lubin A. Spectral analysis of the EEG during waking and sleeping. Electroencephalogr Clin Neurophysiol 1967;23:80.

87. Stepanski E, Salava W, Lamphere J, et al. Experimental sleep fragmentation and sleepiness in normal subjects: a preliminary report. Sleep Res 1984;13:193.

88. Bliwise D, Bliwise NC, Kramer HC, Dement W. Measurement error in visually scored electro physiological data: respiration during sleep. J Neurosci Methods 1984;12:49–56.

89. Caterall JR, Calverley PMA, Shapiro CM, et al. Breathing and oxygenation during sleep are similar in normal men and normal women. Am Rev Respir Dis 1985;132:86–88.

90. Bradley TD, Brown IG, Zamel N, et al. Differences in pharyngeal properties between snorers with predominantly central sleep apnea and those without sleep apnea. Am Rev Respir Dis 1987;135:387–391.

91. West P, Kryger MH. Continuous monitoring of respiratory variables during sleep by microcomputer. Methods Inf Med 1983;22:198–203.

92. Block AJ, Boysen PG, Wynne JW, Hunt LA. Sleep apnea, hypopnea and oxygen de saturation in normal subjects. A strong male predominance. N EnglJ Med 1979;300:513–517.

93. Guilleminault C, Stoohs R, Clerk A, et al. Excessive daytime somnolence in women with abnormal respiratory effort during sleep. Sleep 1993;16:S137–S138.

94. Simantirakis EN, Schiza SI, Marketou ME, et al. Severe bradyar-rhythmias in patients with sleep apnoea: the effect of continuous positive airway pressure treatment: a long-term evaluation using an insertable loop recorder. Eur Heart J 2004;25:1070.
95. Tilkian AG, Guilleminault C, Schroeder JS, et al. Sleep induced apnea syndrome – prevalence of cardiac arrhythmias and their reversal after tracheostomy. Am J Med 1977;63:348.
96. Miller WP. Cardiac arrhythmias and conduction disturbances in the sleep apnea syndrome. Prevalence and significance. Am J Med 1982;73:317.
97. Zwillich C, Devlin T, White D, Douglas N. Bradycardia during sleep apnea. Characteristics and mechanism. J Clin Invest 1982;69:1286.
98. Alonso-Fernandez A, Garcia-Rio F, Racionero MA, et al. Cardiac rhythm disturbances and ST-segment depression episodes in patients with obstructive sleep apnea-hypopnea syndrome and its mecha-nisms. Chest 2005;127:15.
99. Gami AS, Friedman PA, Chung MK, et al. Therapy insight: interac-tions between atrial fibrillation and obstructive sleep apnea. Nat Clin Pract Cardiovasc Med 2005;2:145.
100. Guilleminault C, Connolly SJ, Winkle RA. Cardiac arrhythmia and conduction disturbances during sleep in 400 patients with sleep apnea syndrome. Am J Cardiol 1983;52:490.
101. Burger D, Cantani P, West J. Multidimensional analysis of sleep elec-tro physiological signals. Biol Cybern 1977;26:131–139.
102. Gath I, Bar-on E. Computerized method for scoring of polygraphic sleep recordings. Comput Prog Biomed 1980;1l:217–223.
103. Ray SR, Lee WD, Morgan CD, Airth-Kindree W. Computer sleep stage scoring –an expert system approach. Int J Biomed Comput 1986;19:43–61.
104. Gaillard J-M, Tissot R. Principles of automatic analysis of sleep records with a hybrid system. Comput Biomed Res 1973;6:1–13.
105. Smith JR, Karacan I, Lang M. Automated analysis of human sleep EEG. Wake Sleep 1978;2:75–82.
106. Martens WLJ, Declerck AC, Kums GJTM, Wauquier A. Considerations on a computerized analysis oflong-term polygraphic recordings. In: Stefan H, Burr W, eds. EEG Monitoring. Gustav Fischer, Stuttgart, 1982;265–274.
107. Agnew HW, Webb WB. Measurement of sleep onset by EEG criteria. AmJ EEG Technol 1972;12:127–134.
108. Webb WB. Recording methods and visual scoring criteria of sleep records: comments and recommendations. Percept Mot Skills 1986;62:664–666.
109. Dement WC, Kleitman N. Cyclic variations in EEG during sleep and their relation to eye movements, body motility, and dreaming. Electroencephalogr Clin Neurophysiol 1957;9:673–690.
110. Montplaisir J, Billiard M, Takahashi S, et al. Twenty-four-hour recording in REM-narcoleptics with special reference to nocturnal sleep disruption. Biol Psychiatry 1978;13:73–89.
111. Vogel G. Studies in the psychophysiology of dreams. III. The dreams of narcolepsy. Arch Gen Psychiatry 1960;3:421–428.

112. Kupfer DJ. A psychobiologic marker for primary depressive disease. Biol Psychiatry 1976;1l:159–174.

113. Aserinsky E. The maximal capacity for sleep: rapid eye movement density as an index of sleep satiety. Biol Psychiatry 1969;1:147–159.

114. Sackner MA, Lauda J, Forrest T, Greeneltch D. Periodic sleep apnea: chronic sleep deprivation related to intermittent upper airway obstruction and central nervous system disturbance. Chest 1975;67:164–171.

115. Phillipson EA, Sullivan CE, Read DJ, et al. Ventilatory and waking responses to hypoxia in sleeping dogs. J Appl Physiol 1978;44: 512–520.

116. Phillipson EA, Kozar LF, Rebuck AS, Murphy E. Ventilatory and waking responses to CO_2 in sleeping dogs. Am Rev Respir Dis 1977;115:251–259.

117. Karacan I. The developmental aspect and the effect of certain clinical conditions upon penile erection during sleep. Excerpta Med 1966;150:2356–2359.

118. Parmeggiani PL. Temperature regulation during sleep: a study in homeostasis. In: Orem J, Barnes CD, eds: Physiology in Sleep. Academic, New York, 1980;98–145.

119. Chesson AL Jr, Berry RB, Pack A. Practice parameters for the use of portable monitoring devices in the investigation of suspected obstructive sleep apnea in adults. Sleep 2003;26(7):907–913.

120. Bennett JA, Kinnear WJ. Sleep on the cheap: the role of overnight oximetry in the diagnosis of sleep apnea-hypopnea syndrome. Thorax 1999;54:958–959.

121. Stradling JR, Crosby JH. Predictors and prevalence of obstructive sleep apnea and snoring in 1001 middle aged men. Thorax 1991;46:85–90.

122. Rauscher H, Popp W, Zwick H. Computerized detection of respiratory events during sleep from rapid increases in oxyhemoglobin saturation. Lung 1991;169:335–342.

123. Kripke DF, Ancoli-Israel S, Klauber MR, et al. Prevalence of sleep-disordered breathing in ages 40–64 years: a population-based survey. Sleep 1997;20:65–76.

124. Mooe T, Rabben T, Wiklund U, et al. Sleep-disordered breathing in women: occurrence and association with coronary artery disease. Am J Med 1996;101:251–256.

125. Epstein LJ, Dorlac GR. Cost-effectiveness analysis of nocturnal oximetry as a method of screening for sleep apnea-hypopnea syndrome. Chest 1998;113:97–103.

126. Loube DI, Andrada TF. Comparison of respiratory polysomnographic parameters in matched cohorts of upper airway resistance and obstructive sleep apnea syndrome patients. Chest 1999;115: 1519–1524.

127. Cooper BG, Veale D, Griffiths CJ, et al. Value of nocturnal oxygen saturation as a screening test for sleep apnea. Thorax 1991;46:586–588.

128. Sano K, Nakano H, Ohnishi Y, et al. Screening of sleep apnea-hypopnea syndrome by home pulse oximetry. Nihon Kokyuki Gakkai Zasshi 1998;36:948–952.

129. Ryan PJ, Hilton MF, Boldy DAR, et al. Validation of British Thoracic Society guidelines for the diagnosis of the sleep apnea-hypopnea syndrome: can polysomnography be avoided? Thorax 1995;50:972–975.

130. Deegan PC, McNicholas WT. Predictive value of clinical features for the obstructive sleep apnea syndrome. Eur Respir J 1996;9:117–124.

131. Levy P, Pepin JL, Deschaux-Blanc C, et al. Accuracy of oximetry for detection of respiratory disturbances in sleep apnea syndrome. Chest 1996;109:395–399.

132. Vazquez JC, Tsai WH, Flemons WW, et al. Automated analysis of digital oximetry in the diagnosis of obstructive sleep apnea. Thorax 2000;55:302–307.

133. Williams AJ, Yu G, Santiago S, et al. Screening for sleep apnea using pulse oximetry and a clinical score. Chest 1991;100:631–635.

134. Rauscher H, Popp W, Zwick H. Model for investigating snorers with suspected sleep apnea syndrome. Thorax 1993;48:275–279.

135. Peck T. Waveforms are needed to interpret figures shown by pulse oximeters [letter]. BMJ 1999;318:1353.

136. Redline S, Sanders M. Hypopnea, a floating metric: implications for prevalence, morbidity estimates, and case finding. Sleep 1997;20:1209–1217.

137. Netzer N, Eliasson AH, Netzer C, Kristo DA. Overnight pulse oximetry for sleep-disordered breathing in adults: a review. Chest 2001;120:625–633.

138. Ullmer E, Strobel WM, Soler M. Cheyne-Stokes respiration of obstructive sleep apnea: pattern desaturation [letter]. Respiration 2000;67:203.

139. Calderon-Osuna E, Bernal CC, Gordillo MA, et al. A comparative study with chronic obstructive pulmonary disease with and without obstructive sleep apnea syndrome. Arch Bronchoneumol 1999;35:539–543.

140. Kramer MR, Krivoruk V, Lebzelter J, et al. Quantitative 15 steps exercise oximetry as a marker of disease severity in patients with chronic obstructive pulmonary disease. Isr Med Assoc J 1999;1:165–168.

141. Pradhan PS, Glicklich RE, Winkelman J. Screening for obstructive sleep apnea in patients presenting for snoring surgery. Laryngoscope 1996;106:1393–1397.

142. George CF. Diagnostic techniques in obstructive sleep apnea. Prog Cardiovasc Dis 1999;41:355–366.

143. Gonzalez-Moro JMR, de Lucas Ramos P, Juanes MJS, et al. Usefulness of the visual analysis of night oximetry as a screening method in patients with suspected clinical sleep apnea syndrome. Arch Bronconeumol 1996;32:437–441.

144. Schafer H, Ewig S, Hasper E, et al. Predictive diagnostic value of clinical assessment and nonlaboratory monitoring system recordings in patients with symptoms suggestive of obstructive sleep apnea syndrome. Respiration 1997;64:194–199.

145. Nuber R, Varvrina J, Karrer W. Predictive value of nocturnal pulse oximetry in sleep apnea screening. Schweiz Med Wochenschr Suppl 2000;116:120S–122S.

146. Golpe R, Jiminez A, Carpizo R, et al. Utility of home oximetry as a screening test for patients with moderate to severe symptoms of obstructive sleep apnea. Sleep 1999;22:932–937.

147. Lacassagne L, Didier A, Murris-Espin M, et al. Role of nocturnal oximetry in screening for sleep apnea syndrome in pulmonary medicine: study of 329 patients. Rev Mal Respir 1997;14:201–207.

148. Olson LG, Ambrobetti A, Gyulay SG. Prediction of sleep-disordered breathing by unattended overnight oximetry. J Sleep Res 1999;8:51–55.

149. Brouillette RT, Morielli A, Leimanis A, et al. Nocturnal pulse oximetry as an abbreviated testing modality for pediatric obstructive sleep apnea. Pediatrics 2000;105:405–412.

150. Mahlmeister MJ, Fink JB, Cohen NH. A strategy for reducing costs associated with pulse oximetry in noncritical care areas. Respir Care 1993;38:1005–1013.

151. Chiner E, Signes-Costa J, Arriero JM, et al. Nocturnal oximetry for the diagnosis of the sleep apnea-hypopnea syndrome: a method to reduce the number of polysomnographies? Thorax 1999;54:968–971.

152. Carskadon MA, Dement WC. Cumulative effects of sleep restriction on daytime sleepiness. Psychophysiology 1981;18:107–113.

153. Carskadon MA, Dement WC. Effects of total sleep loss on sleep tendency. Percept Mot Skills 1979;48:495–506.

154. Carskadon MA, Harvey K, Dement WC. Acute restriction of nocturnal sleep in children. Percept Mot Skills 1981;53:103–112.

155. Carskadon MA, Harvey K, Dement WC. Sleep loss in young adolescents. Sleep 1981;4:299–312.

156. Carskadon MA, Dement WC. Sleep loss in elderly volunteers. Sleep 1985;8:207–221.

157. Dement WC, Seidel W, Carskadon M. Daytime alertness, insomnia, and benzodiazepines. Sleep 1982;5:528–545.

158. Lumley M, Roehrs T, Asker D, Zorick F, Roth T. Ethanol and caffeine effects on daytime sleepiness/alertness. Sleep 1987;10:306–312.

159. Roehrs T, Tietz EI, Zorick F, Roth T. Daytime sleepiness and antihistamines. Sleep 1984;7:137–141.

160. Richardson GS, Carskadon MA, Flagg W, van den Hoed J, Dement WC, Mitler MM. Excessive daytime sleepiness in man: multiple sleep latency measurement in narcoleptic and control subjects. Electroencephalogr Clin Neurophysiol 1978;45:621–627.

161. Mitler MM, van den Hoed J, Carskadon MA, et al. REM sleep episodes during the multiple sleep test in narcoleptic patients. Electroencephalogr Clin Neurophysiol 1979;46:479–481.

162. Richardson GS, Carskadon MA, Orav EJ, Dement WC. Circadian variation of sleep tendency in elderly and young adult subjects. Sleep 1982;5:S82–S94.
163. Carskadon MA, Dement WC. Nocturnal determinants of daytime sleepiness. Sleep 1982;5:S73–S81.
164. Hartse K, Roth T, Zorick F. Daytime sleepiness and daytime wakefulness: the effect of instruction. Sleep 1982;5:S107–S118.
165. Carskadon MA. The second decade. In: Guilleminault C, ed. Disorders of Sleeping and Waking: Indications and Techniques. Addison-Wesley, Menlo Park, CA, 1982;99–125.
166. Mitler M. The multiple sleep latency test as an evaluation for excessive somnolence. In: Guilleminault C, ed. Disorders of Sleeping and Waking: Indications and Techniques. Addison-Wesley, Menlo Park, CA, 1982;145–153.
167. Browman C, Gujavarty K, Yolles SF, Mitler MM. Forty-eighthour polysomnographic evaluation of narcolepsy. Sleep 1986;9:183–188.
168. Dement WC, Carskadon MA, Richardson GS. Excessive daytime sleepiness in the sleep apnea syndrome. In: Guilleminault C, Dement WC, eds. Sleep Apnea Syndromes. Alan R. Liss, New York, 1978;23–46.
169. Carskadon MA, Littell WP, Dement WC. Constant routine: alertness, oral body temperature, and performance. Sleep Res 1985;14:293.
170. Van den Hoed J, Kraemer H, Guilleminault C, et al. Disorders of excessive daytime somnolence: polygraphic and clinical data for 100 patients. Sleep 1981;4:23–37.
171. Roth T, Hartse KM, Zorick F, Conway W. Multiple naps and the evaluation of daytime sleepiness in patients with upper airway sleep apnea. Sleep 1980;3:425–439.
172. Carskadon MA, Orav EJ, Dement WC. Evolution of sleep and daytime sleepiness in adolescents. In: Guilleminault C, Lugaresi E, eds. Sleep/Wake Disorders: Natural History, Epidemiology, and Long-Term Evolution. Raven, New York, 1983;201–216.
173. Guilleminault C, Dement W. 235 cases of excessive daytime sleepiness. Neural Sci 1977;31:13–27.
174. Carskadon MA. The role of sleep onset REM periods in narcolepsy. In: Guilleminault C, Dement WC, Passouant P, eds: Narcolepsy. Spectrum, New York, 1976;499–517.
175. Reynolds CF, Coble PA, Kupfer DJ, Holzer BC. Application of the multiple sleep latency test in disorders of excessive sleepiness. Electroencephalogr Clin Neurophysiol 1982;53:443–452.
176. Zorick F, Roehrs T, Koshorek G, et al. Patterns of sleepiness in various disorders of excessive daytime somnolence. Sleep 1982;5:S165–S174.
177. Johns MW. A new method for measuring daytime sleepiness: the Epworth sleepiness scale. Sleep 1991;14:540–545.
178. Berry RB. Sleep Medicine Pearls, First Edition. Hanley & Belfus, Philadelphia, PA, 1999.
179. Hoddes E, Zarone V, Smythe H, et al. Quantification of sleepiness: a new approach. Psychophysiology 1973;10:431–436.

180. The Atlas Task Force of the American Sleep Disorders Association. Recording and scoring leg movements. Sleep 1993;16:749–759.
181. Fleetham J, Ayas N, et al. Canadian Thoracic Society guidelines: diagnosis and treatment of sleep disordered breathing in adults. Can Respir J 2007;13:387–392.
182. Mathur R, Douglas NJ. Frequency of EEG arousals from nocturnal sleep in mormal subjects. Sleep 1995;18:330–333.

Appendix 1: Abbreviations

PFT

ALS	Amyotrophic lateral sclerosis
ARDS	Acute respiratory distress syndrome
ATS	American Thoracic Society
BD	Bronchodilator(s)
BHT	Breath-hold time
BMI	Body mass index
CHF	Congestive heart failure
C_{Ldyn}	Dynamic compliance
C_{Lstat}	Static compliance
CO	Carbon monoxide
CO_2	Carbon dioxide
COPD	Chronic obstructive pulmonary disease
CVA	Cerebrovascular accident
dl	Deciliter
DL_{CO}	Diffusing capacity of carbon monoxide
ERS	European Respiratory Society
ERV	Expiratory reserve volume
FEF	Forced expiratory flow
FET	Forced expiratory time
FEV_1	Forced expiratory volume in the 1st second
FEV_6	Forced expiratory volume in 6 s
FIF	Forced inspiratory flow
FIVC	Forced inspiratory vital capacity
FRC	Functional residual capacity
FV curve	Flow volume curve
FV loop	Flow volume loop
FVC	Forced vital capacity

G_{AW}	Airway conductance
g	Gram
H_2O	Water
He	Helium
Hgb	Hemoglobin
IC	Inspiratory capacity
ILD	Interstitial lung disease
IPF	Idiopathic pulmonary fibrosis
IRV	Inspiratory reserve volume
IVC	Inspiratory vital capacity
MDI	Metered dose inhaler
mg	Milligram
MEP	Maximal expiratory pressure
MI	Myocardial infarction
MIP	Maximal inspiratory pressure
MMEF	Maximal med-expiratory flow
ms	Millisecond
MSD	Musculoskeletal disease
MVV	Maximal voluntary ventilation
N_2	Nitrogen
NMD	Neuromuscular disease
O_2	Oxygen
OSA	Obstructive sleep apnea
P_{atm}, P_B	Atmospheric pressure or barometric pressure
P_{di}	Diaphragmatic pressure
PEF	Peak expiratory flow
P_{es}	Esophageal pressure
PFT	Pulmonary function test
PIF	Peak inspiratory flow
P_IO_2	Partial pressure of inspired oxygen
P_{nas}	Nasal pressure
P_{ga}	Gastric pressure
R_{AW}	Airway resistance
RV	Residual volume
SG_{AW}	Specific airway conductance
SOB	Shortness of breath
SR_{AW}	Specific airway resistance
SVC	Slow vital capacity
TGV (V_{TG})	Thoracic gas volume
TLC	Total lung capacity

V_A	Alveolar volume
VC	Vital capacity
V_{TG}	(TGV) Thoracic gas volume
V_T	Tidal volume
VT curve	Volume time curve
% pred.	Percent predicted

ABG

ABG	Arterial blood gas
AG	Anion gap
AGMA	Anion gap metabolic acidosis
AV malf.	Arteriovenous malformation
BE	Base excess
Cl^-	Chloride
COPD	Chronic obstructive pulmonary disease
F_IO_2	Fractional inspired oxygen
H^+	Proton
$[H^+]$	Hydrogen ion concentration
HCl	Hydrochloric acid
HCO_3^+	Bicarbonate
$[HCO_3^+]$	Bicarbonate concentration
ILD	Interstitial lung disease
K	Constant
kPa	Kilopascal
Na^+	Sodium
NAG	Nonanion gap
NAGMA	Nonanion gap metabolic acidosis
$NaHCO_3$	Sodium bicarbonate
NH_4^+	Ammonium
NH_4Cl	Ammonium chloride
O_2	Oxygen
$P_{(A-a)}O_2$	Alveolar arterial oxygen gradient
P_aCO_2	Partial pressure of arterial carbon dioxide
P_ACO_2	Partial pressure of alveolar carbon dioxide
P_aO_2	Partial pressure of arterial oxygen
P_AO_2	Partial pressure of alveolar oxygen
$P_{atm}O_2$	Partial pressure of atmospheric oxygen
P_{H2O}	Partial pressure of water vapor
P_IO_2	Partial pressure of inspired oxygen

RA	Room air
RQ	Respiratory quotient
RTA	Renal tubular acidosis
S_aO_2	Arterial oxygen saturation
TPN	Total parenteral nutrition
VQ mismatch	Ventilation perfusion mismatch
ΔG	Delta gap

Exercise test

12MWT	12-min walk test
6MWD	6-min walk distance
6MWT	6-min walk test
AT	Anaerobic threshold
BP	Blood pressure
C.O.	Cardiac output
C_aO_2	Arterial oxygen content
CF	Cystic fibrosis
CHF	Congestive heart failure
$C_{\bar{v}}O_2$	Mixed venous oxygen content
DVT	Deep venous thrombosis
ECG	Electrocardiogram
Ft	Foot (Feet)
HR	Heart rate
LVF	Left ventricular failure
MI	Myocardial infarction
PE	Pulmonary embolism
$P_{ET}CO_2$	End-tidal carbon dioxide tension
$P_{ET}O_2$	End-tidal oxygen tension
RR	Respiratory rate
S_pO_2	Arterial Oxygen saturation with pulse oximetry
SV	Stroke volume
$S_{\bar{v}}O_2$	Mixed venous oxygen saturation
V_A	Alveolar volume
V_D	Dead space volume
V_D/V_T	Dead space fraction

$\dot{V}_A$	Alveolar ventilation per minute
$\dot{V}CO_2$	Carbon dioxide production per minute
$\dot{V}_D$	Dead space ventilation per minute
$\dot{V}_D/\dot{V}_E$	Dead space fraction
$\dot{V}E$	Minute ventilation
$\dot{V}O_2$	Oxygen consumption per minute

Diagnostic tests for sleep disorders

AHI	Apnea hypopnea index
AI	Apnea index
COPD	Chronic obstructive pulmonary disease
CPAP	Continuous positive airway pressure
CSA	Central sleep apnea
ECG	Electrocardiography
EEG	Electroencephalography
EMG	Electromyography
EOG	Electrooculography
GERD	Gastroesophageal reflux disease
HI	Hyponea index
Hz	Hertz
LOC	Left outer canthus
MSLT	Multiple sleep latency test
MWT	Maintenance of wakefulness test
NREM	Nonrapid eye movement
ODI	Oxygen desaturation index
OSA	Obstructive sleep apnea
OSAH	Obstructive sleep apnea/hypopnea
PLM-AI	Periodic limb movement arousal index
PLMD	Periodic limb movement disorder
PLM-I	Periodic limb movement index
PSG	Polysomnography
REM	Rapid eye movement
RERA	Respiratory effort-related arousal
RLS	Restless leg syndrome
ROC	Right outer canthus
SE	Sleep efficiency
SEM	Slow rolling eye movement
SOL	Sleep onset latency

S_pO_2 Oxygen saturation by pulse oximetry
SPT   Sleep period time
SSRI   Selective serotonin reuptake inhibitors
SVT   Supraventricular tachycardia

TIB   Time in bed
TST   Total sleep time

UARS   Upper airway resistance syndrome

V_T Tidal volume
VT   Ventricular tachycardia

WASO   Wake after sleep onset

Appendix 2: Normal Values

PFT Normal Values (ATS) – Apply Mainly to Young and Middle Ages

FVC	80–120 (% Pred.)
FEV_1	80–120
FEV_1/FVC ratio	80–120
FEF_{25-75}	>65% pred. but can be as low as 55%
FEF_{25-75}/FVC ratio	>0.66 (more accurate)
TLC	80–120
FRC	75–120
RV	75–120
DL_{CO}	80–120
MEP	>90 cmH_2O
MIP	<–70 cmH_2O
Supine FVC	Within 10% of the sitting value; >30% drop suggests diaphragmatic paralysis

PFT Absolute Figures (for an Average Young Adult Male; Listed in a Decreasing Order)

TLC	6 L
FVC	5 L
FEV_1	4 L
FRC	3 L
ERV	1–2 L
RV	1–2 L
DL_{CO}	25 ml/min/mmHg

PFT Grading of Severity of Obstructive and Restrictive Disorders

(A) Grading of severity of any spirometric abnormality based on FEV_1:
- After determining the pattern to be obstructive, restrictive, or mixed, FEV_1 is used to grade severity:

Mild	FEV_1 > 70 (% pred.)
Moderate	60–69
Moderately severe	50–59
Severe	35–49
Very severe	<35

(B) Traditional method of grading the severity of obstructive and restrictive disorders:
  • Obstructive disorder (based on FEV_1) – ratio < 0.7

May be a physiologic variant	FEV_1 = 100 (% pred.)
Mild	70–100
Moderate	60–69
Moderately severe	50–59
Severe	35–49
Very severe	<35

  • Restrictive disorder (based on TLC, preferred)

Mild	TLC > 70 (% pred.)
Moderate	60–69
Severe	<60

  • Restrictive disorder (based on FVC, in case no lung volume study is available)

Mild	FVC > 70 (% pred.)
Moderate	60–69
Moderately severe	50–59
Severe	35–49
Very severe	<35

ABG NORMAL VALUES

pH	7.35–7.45
P_aCO_2	35–45 mmHg
P_aO_2	>80 mmHg
HCO_3	21–26 mmol/L (consider it 24)
BE	0 to –2 mmol/L
S_aO_2	>95%
AG	10 ± 4
$P_{(A-a)}O_2$	<15 (increases with age)

EXERCISE TEST NORMAL VALUES

$\dot{V}O_2$max	83%
AT	>40% of predicted Vo_2max
BP	<220/90
O_2 pulse	>80% predicted
HR max	(220 – age) ± 15 beats or >90% of that predicted for age
HR reserve	0 ± 15 beats or <15 beats/min
RQ (at peak exercise)	≤1
RR max	<60 breaths/min
Ventilatory reserve	>11 L/min
Breathing reserve	<85%
$\dot{V}E/\dot{V}CO_2$ (at AT)	<34
$\dot{V}E/\dot{V}O_2$ (at AT)	<31
V_D/V_T (at peak exercise)	0.2–0.3

Appendix 3: Conversions

TO CONVERT FROM KILOPASCAL TO MMHG:
Multiply by 7.5

CONVERTING PH TO [H⁺]:
- When pH is within 7.30–7.50
  - pH of 7.40 ↔ [H⁺] = 40 nmol/L.
  - Then *increasing* or decreasing pH by 0.01 is equivalent to *decreasing* or increasing [H⁺] by 1 nmol/L (remember that [H⁺] changes in the opposite direction of pH; for instance, acidosis decreases pH and increases [H⁺]).
  - So if pH is 7.35, then [H⁺] will equal 40 + 5 = 45 nmol/L.
- When pH is outside that range (this can be applied within that range too):
  - pH of 7.00 ↔ [H⁺] = 100 nmol/L.
  - Then every *increase* or decrease of pH by 0.10 is equivalent to *multiplying* or dividing [H⁺] by 0.8.
  - So if pH is 7.10, then [H⁺] will equal 100 × 0.8 = 80 nmol/L.
  - If pH is 7.20, then [H⁺] will equal 100 × 0.8 × 0.8 = 64 nmol/l.
  - If pH is 7.40, then [H⁺] = $100 \times 0.8^4 = 40$.
  - If pH is 6.80, then [H⁺] = 100/(0.8 × 0.8) = 156.
- If you do not want to bother yourself with these boring calculations, the following table can be of help:

pH	[H⁺]	pH	[H⁺]
7.00	100	7.35	45
7.05	89	7.40	40
7.10	79	7.45	35
7.15	71	7.50	32
7.20	63	7.55	28
7.25	56	7.60	25
7.30	50	7.65	22

ESTIMATING F_IO_2 WHEN USING SUPPLEMENTAL O_2

The information provided in this section is acquired from "American Heart Association. Advanced Cardiac Life Support (ACLS) provider manual, 2001" and represents just a rough estimation of the F_IO_2.

- *Breathing through nasal cannula*: Consider F_IO_2 at RA (20%), then each liter of O_2 corresponds to 4% increment in F_IO_2 over the 20%:
  - 1 L   24%
  - 2 L   28%
  - 3 L   32%
  - 4 L   36%
  - 5 L   40%
  - 6 L   44%
- *Breathing through a face mask*: 6–10 l of O_2 increases F_IO_2 to ~60%.
- *Breathing through a face mask with O_2 reservoir (nonrebreather mask)*: each liter of O_2 (starting from 6 l) corresponds to 10% increment in F_IO_2 (starting from 60%).
  - 6 L   60%
  - 7 L   70%
  - 8 L   80%
  - 9 L   90%
  - 10–15 L ~100%
- *Breathing through a venturi mask*: gives a more accurate estimation of F_IO_2 (amount of F_IO_2 delivered is written on the mask itself).

Index

RA	Room air
RQ	Respiratory quotient
RTA	Renal tubular acidosis
S_aO_2	Arterial oxygen saturation
TPN	Total parenteral nutrition
VQ mismatch	Ventilation perfusion mismatch
ΔG	Delta gap

Exercise test

12MWT	12-min walk test
6MWD	6-min walk distance
6MWT	6-min walk test
AT	Anaerobic threshold
BP	Blood pressure
C.O.	Cardiac output
C_aO_2	Arterial oxygen content
CF	Cystic fibrosis
CHF	Congestive heart failure
$C_{\bar{v}}O_2$	Mixed venous oxygen content
DVT	Deep venous thrombosis
ECG	Electrocardiogram
Ft	Foot (Feet)
HR	Heart rate
LVF	Left ventricular failure
MI	Myocardial infarction
PE	Pulmonary embolism
$P_{ET}CO_2$	End-tidal carbon dioxide tension
$P_{ET}O_2$	End-tidal oxygen tension
RR	Respiratory rate
S_PO_2	Arterial Oxygen saturation with pulse oximetry
SV	Stroke volume
$S_{\bar{v}}O_2$	Mixed venous oxygen saturation
V_A	Alveolar volume
V_D	Dead space volume
V_D/V_T	Dead space fraction

V_A	Alveolar volume
VC	Vital capacity
V_{TG}	(TGV) Thoracic gas volume
V_T	Tidal volume
VT curve	Volume time curve
% pred.	Percent predicted

ABG	
ABG	Arterial blood gas
AG	Anion gap
AGMA	Anion gap metabolic acidosis
AV malf.	Arteriovenous malformation
BE	Base excess
Cl-	Chloride
COPD	Chronic obstructive pulmonary disease
F_1O_2	Fractional inspired oxygen
H+	Proton
[H+]	Hydrogen ion concentration
HCl	Hydrochloric acid
HCO_3^+	Bicarbonate
$[HCO_3^+]$	Bicarbonate concentration
ILD	Interstitial lung disease
K	Constant
kPa	Kilopascal
Na+	Sodium
NAG	Nonanion gap
NAGMA	Nonanion gap metabolic acidosis
$NaHCO_3$	Sodium bicarbonate
NH_4^+	Ammonium
NH_4Cl	Ammonium chloride

O_2	Oxygen
$P_{(A-a)}O_2$	Alveolar arterial oxygen gradient
P_aCO_2	Partial pressure of arterial carbon dioxide
P_ACO_2	Partial pressure of alveolar carbon dioxide
P_aO_2	Partial pressure of arterial oxygen
P_AO_2	Partial pressure of alveolar oxygen
$P_{atm}O_2$	Partial pressure of atmospheric oxygen
P_{H2O}	Partial pressure of water vapor
P_1O_2	Partial pressure of inspired oxygen

WITHDRAWN

CPSIA information can be obtained at www.ICGtesting.com
Printed in the USA
244392LV00010B/6/P

9 781848 822306